GUIDELINES FOR HUMAN EMBRYONIC STEM CELL RESEARCH

Committee on Guidelines for Human Embryonic Stem Cell Research

Board on Life Sciences
Division on Earth and Life studies

Board on Health Sciences Policy
Institute of Medicine

NATIONAL RESEARCH COUNCIL *AND*
INSTITUTE OF MEDICINE
OF THE NATIONAL ACADEMIES

THE NATIONAL ACADEMIES PRESS
Washington, D.C.
www.nap.edu

THE NATIONAL ACADEMIES PRESS 500 Fifth Street, NW   Washington, DC 20001

NOTICE: The project that is the subject of this report was approved by the Governing Board of the National Research Council, whose members are drawn from the councils of the National Academy of Sciences, the National Academy of Engineering, and the Institute of Medicine. The members of the committee responsible for the report were chosen for their special competences and with regard for appropriate balance.

This material is based on work supported by the National Academies, the Ellison Medical Foundation, and the Greenwall Foundation.

Library of Congress Cataloging-in-Publication Data

Guidelines for human embryonic stem cell research / Board on Life Sciences, National Research Council, Board on Health Sciences Policy, Institute of Medicine.
    p. cm.
 Includes bibliographical references and index.
  ISBN 0-309-09653-7 (pbk.) — ISBN 0-309-55024-6 (pdf) 1. Embryonic stem cells—Research. 2. Human embryo—Research. I. National Research Council (U.S.). Board on Life Sciences. II. National Research Council (U.S.). Board on Health Sciences Policy.
  QH588.S83G85 2005
  616'.02774—dc22

2005016338

Additional copies of this report are available from the National Academies Press, 500 Fifth Street, NW, Lockbox 285, Washington, DC 20055; (800) 624-6242 or (202) 334-3313 (in the Washington metropolitan area); Internet, http://www.nap.edu.

Cover: A cluster of motor neurons and neural fibers derived from human embryonic stem cells in the lab of University of Wisconsin-Madison stem cell researcher and neurodevelopmental biologist Su-Chun Zhang. The motor neurons are shown in red; neural fibers appear green and the blue specks indicate DNA in cell nuclei. These motor neurons were developed from one of James Thomson's original human embryonic stem cell lines. Copyright for the photograph is held by the University of Wisconsin's Board of Regents.

THE NATIONAL ACADEMIES
Advisers to the Nation on Science, Engineering, and Medicine

The **National Academy of Sciences** is a private, nonprofit, self-perpetuating society of distinguished scholars engaged in scientific and engineering research, dedicated to the furtherance of science and technology and to their use for the general welfare. Upon the authority of the charter granted to it by the Congress in 1863, the Academy has a mandate that requires it to advise the federal government on scientific and technical matters. Dr. Ralph J. Cicerone is president of the National Academy of Sciences.

The **National Academy of Engineering** was established in 1964, under the charter of the National Academy of Sciences, as a parallel organization of outstanding engineers. It is autonomous in its administration and in the selection of its members, sharing with the National Academy of Sciences the responsibility for advising the federal government. The National Academy of Engineering also sponsors engineering programs aimed at meeting national needs, encourages education and research, and recognizes the superior achievements of engineers. Dr. Wm. A. Wulf is president of the National Academy of Engineering.

The **Institute of Medicine** was established in 1970 by the National Academy of Sciences to secure the services of eminent members of appropriate professions in the examination of policy matters pertaining to the health of the public. The Institute acts under the responsibility given to the National Academy of Sciences by its congressional charter to be an adviser to the federal government and, upon its own initiative, to identify issues of medical care, research, and education. Dr. Harvey V. Fineberg is president of the Institute of Medicine.

The **National Research Council** was organized by the National Academy of Sciences in 1916 to associate the broad community of science and technology with the Academy's purposes of furthering knowledge and advising the federal government. Functioning in accordance with general policies determined by the Academy, the Council has become the principal operating agency of both the National Academy of Sciences and the National Academy of Engineering in providing services to the government, the public, and the scientific and engineering communities. The Council is administered jointly by both Academies and the Institute of Medicine. Dr. Ralph J. Cicerone and Dr. Wm. A. Wulf are chair and vice chair, respectively, of the National Research Council.

www.national-academies.org

Preface

We are pleased to offer our committee's report on guidelines for human embryonic stem cell research. This report and its recommendations are the result of many hours of committee meetings as well as a public workshop. During those sessions we heard from many dedicated and talented people who represent a wide range of views. We have tried to take these diverse perspectives into account in a report that mirrors the seriousness with which we have reflected upon them. Our task was made more difficult and also more significant by events in the worlds of science and public affairs, which altered the terrain even as we explored it. All of us on the committee have appreciated the opportunity to be part of this important and timely effort.

Great possibilities for improvements in human health are offered by research using human stem cells, both adult and embryonic. Like many scientific advances, these technologies raise questions about balancing the evident promise against the potential for inappropriate application. In the case of embryonic stem cell research, there are differing opinions within our society about the relative merits and risks of various approaches and there are philosophical differences about what is or is not appropriate. Some believe strongly that we should not turn away from the promise that embryonic stem cells will provide new therapeutic advances. Others believe that the derivation and application of human embryonic stem cells will undermine the dignity of human life. These disparate views are deeply and sincerely held and must be considered as we move forward in advancing this research. Some of the qualms arise from unfamiliarity and the "shock of the new," but others arise from concerns about the nature of human life, about ethical treatment of reproductive materials and about exploitation of donors of such materials. Those ethical concerns need to be balanced against the duty to provide the best medical care possible, enhancing the quality of life and alleviating suffering for many people. The challenge to our society is to achieve that balance.

Scientific inquiry should not proceed unfettered, without consideration for the ethical and public policy imperatives of the society in which it operates. On the other hand, concerns about potential ethical complexities should be cause for judicious oversight and regulation, not necessarily for prohibition. Our democratic society should be capable of entertaining challenges to familiar beliefs and adapting to new conditions without yielding on its fundamental values. We believe that it is possible to do so, that human dignity will be enhanced, rather than diminished, by the great project of addressing the suffering that attends illness. Freedom of inquiry and a confident attitude toward the future are at the heart of America's civic philosophy, in which the freedom to explore controversial ideas is celebrated rather than suppressed. That is one reason that our country's scientific establishment is the envy of the world, a source of our inventive energy that was celebrated by Thomas Jefferson who wrote, "Liberty is the great parent of science and of virtue; and a nation will be great in both in proportion as it is free."

In that spirit we offer this report.

Richard O. Hynes
Jonathan D. Moreno
Co-chairs, Committee on Guidelines for
Human Embryonic Stem Cell Research

Acknowledgments

Like all National Academies reports, this one is the result of the contributions of many people. First, we sincerely thank all the speakers who participated in our workshop, "Guidelines for Human Embryonic Stem Cell Research," on October 12-13, 2004. A workshop agenda and a list of the workshop speakers with their biographies are included in Appendix C. Without their input, this report would not have been possible.

Second, we would like to thank the Ellison Medical Foundation and the Greenwall Foundation for their financial support of this activity.

This report has been reviewed in draft form by persons chosen for their diverse perspectives and technical expertise in accordance with procedures approved by the National Research Council's Report Review Committee. The purpose of this independent review is to provide candid and critical comments that will assist the institution in making its published report as sound as possible and to ensure that the report meets institutional standards of objectivity, evidence, and responsiveness to the study charge. The review comments and draft manuscript remain confidential to protect the integrity of the deliberative process. We wish to thank the following for their review of this report:

Alexander Capron, World Health Organization
Mark Fishman, Novartis
Linda Giudice, Stanford School of Medicine
Virginia Hinshaw, University of California, Davis
Brigid Hogan, Duke University
Bernard Lo, University of California, San Francisco

Michael Manganiello, Christopher Reeve Foundation
Doug Melton, Harvard University
Catherine Racowsky, Brigham and Women's Hospital
Laura Robbins, Weill Cornell Medical College
John Robertson, University of Texas Law School
Harold Shapiro, Princeton University
Harold Varmus, Memorial Sloan-Kettering Cancer Center
LeRoy Walters, Georgetown University

Although the reviewers listed above have provided many constructive comments and suggestions, they were not asked to endorse the conclusions or recommendations nor did they see the final draft of the report before its release. The review of this report was overseen by Floyd E. Bloom, Scripps Research Institute, and William H. Danforth, Washington University. Appointed by the National Research Council, they were responsible for making certain that an independent examination of this report was carried out in accordance with institutional procedures and that all review comments were carefully considered. Responsibility for the final content of this report rests entirely with the authoring committee and the institution.

Finally, we wish to acknowledge Dr. Kathi Hanna, our superb science writer, and the National Research Council staff (Fran Sharples, Robin Schoen, Matt McDonough, and Norman Grossblatt) for their thorough, thoughtful, and efficient assistance with all aspects of the preparation of this report.

Contents

Summary

This report provides guidelines for the responsible practice of human embryonic stem (hES) cell research. Since 1998, the volume of research being conducted using hES cells has expanded primarily using private funds because of restrictions on the use of federal funds for such research. Although privately funded hES cell research is currently subject to many of the same oversight requirements as other biomedical research, given restricted federal involvement and the absence of federal regulations specifically designed for hES cell research, there is a perception that the field is unregulated. More accurately, there is a patchwork of existing regulations that are applicable to hES cell research, many of which were not designed with this research specifically in mind, and there are gaps in how well they cover hES cell research. In addition, hES cell research touches on many ethical, legal, scientific, and policy issues that are of concern to the public. The guidelines, which are set forth in the final chapter of the report, are intended to enhance the integrity of privately funded hES cell research both in the public's perception and in actuality by encouraging responsible practices in the conduct of that research. The body of the report provides the background and rationale for the choices involved in formulating the guidelines.

In 1998, James Thomson and co-workers became the first scientists to derive and successfully culture human embryonic stem cells (hES cells) from a human blastocyst, an early human embryo of approximately 200 cells, donated by a couple who had completed infertility treatments. Although ES cells had been derived from mouse blastocysts since 1981, this achievement with human cells was significant because of its implications for improved health. The dual capacity of hES cells for self-renewal and for differentiation into repair cells offers great potential for understanding disease development and progression, for regenerative medicine, and for targeted drug development.

In addition to that research accomplishment, the cloning of Dolly the sheep in 1997 using a technique called somatic cell nuclear transfer (SCNT) or, more simply, nuclear transfer (NT) provided a means of generating ES cells with defined genetic makeup. hES cell preparations could potentially be produced by using NT to replace the nucleus of a human oocyte, trigger development, and then isolate hES cells at the blastocyst stage. The advantage of using NT to derive hES cells is that the nuclear genomes of the resulting hES cells would be identical with those of the donors of the somatic cells. One obvious benefit is that this would avoid the problem of rejection if cells generated from the hES cells were to be transplanted into the donor. A more immediate benefit would be facilitation of a wide array of experiments to explore the underpinnings of genetic disease and possible forms of amelioration and cure. Some such experiments will not be possible using hES cells derived from blastocysts generated by *in vitro* fertilization (IVF), in which the nuclear genomes are not defined. Although the promise of using NT for such research is as yet unrealized, most researchers believe that it will be a critical source of both important knowledge and clinical resources. Use of NT for biomedical research, as distinct from its use to create a human being, has been considered by several advisory groups to be ethically acceptable provided that such research is conducted according to established safeguards against misuse and has undergone proper prior review. However, there is nearly universal agreement that use of NT to attempt to produce a child should not be allowed at present. The medical risks are unacceptable, and many people have additional objections to using this procedure for attempts at human procreation.

hES cells currently can be derived from three sources: blastocysts remaining after infertility treatments and donated for research, blastocysts produced from donated gametes (oocytes and sperm), and the products of NT. Ethical concerns about those sources of hES cells—combined with fears that the use of NT for research could lead to its use to produce a child—have fostered much public discussion and debate. In addition, concern has been expressed about whether and how to restrict the production of human/nonhuman chimeras in hES cell research. Research using chimeras will be valuable in understanding the etiology and progression of human disease and in testing new drugs, and will be necessary in preclinical testing of hES cells and their derivatives.

Because there is widespread agreement in the international scientific community about the potential value of hES cell research, the volume of this research has expanded since 1998, despite restrictions in the United States. First, federal legislation forbids the use of federal monies for any research that destroys an embryo; this effectively prevents any use of federal funds to derive hES cells from blastocysts. Second, research with established hES cell lines is limited by a policy announced by President George W. Bush in 2001 that restricts federal funding to research conducted with specific federally approved hES cell lines already in existence before August 9, 2001. Despite the restricted use of federal funds for research of this kind, the derivation of new cell lines is proceeding legally in the private sector and in academic settings with private funds except in those states where such research has been partially or totally banned.

Privately funded hES cell research is subject to some regulation or other constraints primarily through human subjects protections regulations, limits placed on licensees by the holders of NT and hES cell patents, animal care and use regulations, state laws, and self-imposed institutional guidelines at companies and universities that are now doing or contemplating this research. Those aiming to produce biological therapies are also subject to Food and Drug Administration (FDA) regulation. However, because of the absence of federal funding for most current hES cell research, some standard protections may be lacking, and the implementation of protections is not uniform across the country. Moreover, the techniques for deriving the cells do not yet amount to fully developed standard research tools, and the development of any therapeutic application remains some years away. The best way to move forward with hES cell research in pursuit of scientific goals and new therapies is with a set of guidelines to which the U.S. scientific community will adhere. Heightened oversight also is essential to assure the public that such research is being conducted in an ethical manner.

Established criteria for deriving hES cell lines and reviewing research will help to ensure that the derivation, storage, and maintenance of cells meet a standard set of requirements for provenance and ethical review. Because not all scientists want or have the resources to derive new hES cell lines, the ability to share cell lines will create greater access for qualified scientists to participate in stem cell research. The tradition of sharing materials and results with colleagues speeds scientific progress and symbolizes to the nonscientific world that the goals of science are to expand knowledge and to improve the human condition. One key reason for the remarkable success of science since its emergence in modern form—besides the application of the scientific method itself—is the communal nature of scientific activity.

STATEMENT OF COMMITTEE TASK

The National Academies initiated this project to develop guidelines for hES cell research to advance the science in a responsible manner. The Committee on Guidelines for Human Embryonic Stem Cell Research was asked to develop guidelines to encourage responsible practices in hES cell research—regardless of source of funding—including the use and derivation of new stem cell lines derived from surplus blastocysts, from blastocysts produced with donated gametes, or from blastocysts produced using NT. The guidelines take ethical and legal concerns into account and encompass the basic science and health science policy issues related to the development and use of hES cells for research and eventual therapeutic purposes, such as

1. Recruitment of donors of blastocysts, gametes, or somatic cells including medical exclusion criteria, informed consent, the use of financial incentives, risks associated with oocyte retrieval, confidentiality, and the interpretation of genetic information that is developed from studies with these materials and that might have importance to the donors.
2. The characterization of stem cells for purposes of standardization and for validation of results.
3. The safe handling and storage of blastocysts and stem cell material and conditions for transfer of such material among laboratories.
4. Prerequisites to hES cell research (such as examination of alternative approaches), appropriate uses of hES cells in research or therapy and limitations on the use of hES cells.
5. Safeguards against misuse.

To conduct its work, the committee surveyed the current state of science in this field and probable pending developments, reviewed the policy and ethical issues posed by the research, examined professional and international regulations and guidelines that relate to hES cell research, and conducted a 2-day workshop to hear representatives of many scientific, ethical, and public policy perspectives. The committee did not revisit the debate about whether hES cell research should be pursued; it assumed that both hES cell and adult stem cell research would continue in parallel with federal and nonfederal funding.

WHAT THE GUIDELINES COVER

The guidelines are intended for the use of the scientific community, including researchers in university, industry, or other private-sector organizations. They cover all derivations of hES cell lines and all research using hES cells derived from

1. Blastocysts made for reproductive purposes and later obtained for research from IVF clinics.
2. Blastocysts made specifically for research using IVF.
3. Somatic cell nuclear transfer (NT) into oocytes.

The guidelines do not cover research with nonhuman stem cells. In addition, many but not all of the guidelines and concerns addressed in this report are common to other areas of human stem cell research, such as research with adult stem cells, fetal stem cells, or embryonic germ cells derived from fetal tissue. Institutions and investigators conducting research with such materials should consider which individual provisions of the guidelines set forth in this report are relevant to their research.

The guidelines do not apply to reproductive uses of NT, which are addressed in the 2002 report *Scientific and Medical Aspects of Human Reproductive Cloning*, in which the National Academies stated that "Human reproductive cloning should not now be practiced. It is dangerous and likely to fail." Although these guidelines do not specifically address attempts to use NT for reproductive purposes, it continues to be the view of the National Academies that such attempts should not be conducted at this time.

MAJOR RECOMMENDATIONS

This summary provides the major recommendations made by the committee, each of which supports an operational aspect of the guidelines presented in Chapter 6. Central to the recommendations is a dual system of oversight at the institutional and national levels. This system of oversight will ensure that the highest ethical, legal, and scientific standards are met in the derivation, storage, and use of hES cells in research.

Institutional Oversight of hES Cell Research

The ethical and legal concerns involved in hES cell research make increased local oversight by research institutions appropriate. Because of the complexity and novelty of many of the issues involved in hES cell research, the committee believes that all research institutions conducting hES cell research should create special review bodies to oversee this emerging field of research. Such committees will be responsible for ensuring that all applicable regulatory requirements are met and that hES cell research is conducted in accordance with the guidelines set forth in this report.

To provide local oversight of all issues related to derivation and research use of hES cell lines and to facilitate education of investigators involved in hES cell research, all institutions conducting hES cell research should establish an Embryonic Stem Cell Research Oversight (ESCRO) committee. The committee should include representatives of the public and persons with expertise in developmental biology, stem cell research, molecular biology, assisted reproduction, and ethical and legal issues in hES cell research. The committee will not substitute for an Institutional Review Board but rather will provide an additional level of review and scrutiny warranted by the complex issues raised by hES cell research. The committee will also review basic hES cell research using preexisting anonymous cell lines that does not require consideration by an Institutional Review Board.

The ESCRO committee will assist investigators in assessing which regulations might apply to proposed research activities. The committee could serve as a clearinghouse for hES cell research proposals and could assist investigators in identifying the types and levels of review required for a given protocol. For example, the creation of a chimera might involve both an Institutional Review Board (IRB), if cells are to be obtained from human donors for research, and an Institutional Animal Care and Use Committee (IACUC), if animals are to be used in the research. In some instances, Institutional Biosafety Committees (IBCs) and radiation safety committees might also have roles to play in research review. If hES cell research involves potential clinical applications (such as development of products to be tested in humans), FDA regulations will apply. However, care should be taken that the ESCRO committee does not duplicate or interfere with the proper functions of an IRB or other existing institutional committee. The functions of IRBs and ESCRO committees are distinct and should not be confused.

One particularly important aspect of regulatory compliance for hES cell research deals with protection of donors of blastocysts and gametes. Laboratory research that uses hES cells is generally not subject to federal regulations governing research with human subjects unless it involves personally identifiable information about the cell line's progenitors. In general, research institutions are likely already to have rules in place for research involving other biological tissues, and hES cell research, like any other form of biological or biomedical research, would be covered by these rules and in many cases will not require further review. In the case of hES cell research, however, it will be critically important for investigators and institutions to know the provenance of hES cell lines, particularly if the cell lines are imported from another institution. That would include obtaining an assurance that the process by which the cells were obtained was approved by an IRB to ensure that donors provided voluntary informed consent and that risks were minimized.

> **Through its Embryonic Stem Cell Research Oversight committee, each research institution should ensure that the provenance of hES cells is documented. Documentation should include evidence that the procurement process was approved by an Institutional Review Board to ensure adherence to the basic ethical and legal principles of informed consent and protection of confidentiality.**

The second role of ESCRO committees is to review research proposals that involve particularly sensitive kinds of research, including all proposals to generate additional hES cell lines by any means. The vast majority of *in vitro* experiments using already derived hES cell lines are unlikely to raise serious ethical issues, and will require minimal review. Some research with hES cells, such as the creation of human/nonhuman chimeras, will need more extensive review.

Other types of studies should not be permitted at this time (such as implantation of embryos or cells into a human uterus or breeding of any interspecies chimera). Still others warrant careful consideration, including research in which identifying information about the donors is available or becomes known to the investigator and experiments involving implantation of hES cells or human neural progenitor cells into nonhuman animals. Because of the sensitive nature of some aspects of hES cell research, it is critical that the scientific community propose and implement limits on what is to be allowed and provide clear guidance on which research activities require greater scrutiny (as discussed in the full report). Thus, a primary activity of ESCRO committees will be to ensure that inappropriate research is not conducted and that sensitive research is well justified (as explained in the full report) and subject to appropriate additional oversight. Oversight will in many instances conform to a higher standard than required by existing laws or regulations. ESCRO committees should have suitable scientific and ethical expertise to conduct their own reviews and should have the resources to coordinate the various other reviews that may be required for a particular protocol. A pre-existing committee could serve the functions of the ESCRO committee provided that it has the recommended expertise to perform the various roles described in this report.

Embryonic Stem Cell Research Oversight (ESCRO) committees or their equivalents should divide research proposals into three categories in setting limits on research and determining the requisite level of oversight:

(a) Research that is permissible after notification of the research institution's ESCRO committee and completion of the reviews mandated by current requirements. Purely *in vitro* hES cell research with pre-existing coded or anonymous hES cell lines in general is permissible provided that notice of the research, documentation of the provenance of the cell lines, and evidence of compliance with any required Institutional Review Board, Institutional Animal Care and Use Committee, Institutional Biosafety Committee, or other mandated reviews, is provided to the ESCRO committee or other body designated by the investigator's institution.

(b) Research that is permissible only after additional review and approval by an ESCRO committee or other equivalent body designated by the investigator's institution.
  (i) The ESCRO committee should evaluate all requests for permission to attempt derivation of new hES cell lines from donated blastocysts, from *in vitro* fertilized oocytes, or by nuclear transfer. The scientific rationale for the need to generate new hES cell lines, by whatever means, should be clearly presented, and the basis for the numbers of blastocysts or oocytes needed should be justified. Such requests should be accompanied by evidence of Institutional Review Board approval of the procurement process.
  (ii) All research involving the introduction of hES cells into nonhuman animals at any stage of embryonic, fetal, or postnatal development should be reviewed by the ESCRO committee. Particular attention should be paid to the probable pattern and effects of differentiation and integration of the human cells into the nonhuman animal tissues.
  (iii) Research in which personally identifiable information about the donors of the blastocysts, gametes, or somatic cells from which the hES cells were

derived is readily ascertainable by the investigator also requires ESCRO committee review and approval.

(c) **Research that should not be permitted at this time.**
(i) **Research involving *in vitro* culture of any intact human embryo, regardless of derivation method, for longer than 14 days or until formation of the primitive streak begins, whichever occurs first.**
(ii) **Research in which hES cells are introduced into nonhuman primate blastocysts or in which any embryonic stem cells are introduced into human blastocysts.**
(iii) **No animal into which hES cells have been introduced at any stage of development should be allowed to breed.**

Because stem cell research is subject to a greater degree of public interest and scrutiny than most other kinds of laboratory research, the committee recommends that each institution should maintain through its ESCRO committee a registry of hES cell lines in use and of investigators working in this field and descriptive information on the types of hES cell research in which they are engaged. The purposes of such a registry include facilitating distribution of educational information in light of evolving ethical, legal, or regulatory issues and enabling the institution to respond to public inquiry about the extent of its involvement in hES cell research.

ADDITIONAL RECOMMENDATIONS

The committee makes several additional recommendations pertaining to the need for IRB review of procurement procedures, the need for voluntary informed consent free of inducements, adherence to standards of clinical care, and compliance with all applicable federal regulations. Those recommendations are summarized here.

Review of the Procurement Process

Research involving hES cells will require access to human oocytes and embryos, necessitating some interaction between oocyte and blastocyst donors and people or institutions seeking to procure these materials for use in hES cell research. Individuals and couples who voluntarily and with full information donate somatic cells, gametes, or blastocysts for hES cell research should be assured that their donation is made for meritorious research and that all efforts will be made by those responsible for handling, storing, and using cell lines to protect donor confidentiality. IRB review of the procurement process, combined with a full informed consent process before donation, will facilitate the ethical conduct of this research.

Regardless of the source of funding and the applicability of federal regulations, an Institutional Review Board or its equivalent should review the procurement of gametes, blastocysts, or somatic cells for the purpose of generating new hES cell lines, including the procurement of blastocysts in excess of clinical need from infertility clinics, blastocysts made through *in vitro* fertilization specifically for research purposes, and oocytes, sperm, and somatic cells donated for development of hES cell lines through nuclear transfer.

Informed Consent of Donors

The donors of sperm, oocytes, or somatic cells used to make blastocysts for research are themselves rarely the subject of the research. Nevertheless, the physical interaction needed to obtain the materials brings them under the purview of the human subjects protections system, and IRB review is required. Thus, their fully informed and voluntary consent is required before such research use.

Institutional Review Boards may not waive the requirement for obtaining informed consent from any person whose somatic cells, gametes, or blastocysts are used in hES cell research.

When donor gametes have been used in the *in vitro* fertilization process, resulting blastocysts may not be used for research without consent of all gamete donors.

In addition to ensuring voluntary informed consent of all donors, there should be no financial incentives in the solicitation or donation of blastocysts, gametes, or somatic cells for research purposes. Nonfinancial incentives also should be avoided. For example, a donor's decision should not be influenced by anticipated personal medical benefits or by concerns about the quality of later care. Thus, a potential donor should be informed that there is no obligation to make such a donation, that no personal benefit will accrue as a result of the decision to donate (except in cases of autologous transplantation), and that no penalty will result from a decision to refuse to donate.

To facilitate autonomous choice, decisions related to the production of embryos for infertility treatment should be free of the influence of investigators who propose to derive or use hES cells in research. Whenever it is practicable, the attending physician responsible for the infertility treatment and the investigator deriving or proposing to use hES cells should not be the same person.

No cash or in kind payments may be provided for donating blastocysts in excess of clinical need for research purposes.

Women who undergo hormonal induction to generate oocytes specifically for research purposes (such as for nuclear transfer) should be reimbursed only for direct expenses incurred as a result of the procedure, as determined by an Institutional Review Board. No cash or in kind payments should be provided for donating oocytes for research purposes. Similarly, no payments should be made for donations of sperm for research purposes or of somatic cells for use in nuclear transfer.

This recommendation should not be interpreted as a commentary on commercial IVF practices, but as a narrow policy position specifically with respect to hES cell research. Furthermore, as with all the policies recommended by the committee, this policy should be regularly reviewed and reconsidered as the field matures and the experiences under other policies can be evaluated.

It is widely accepted that, whenever possible, donors' decisions to dispose of their blastocysts should be made separately from their decisions to donate them for research. Potential donors should be allowed to provide blastocysts for research only if they have decided to have those blastocysts discarded instead of donating them to another couple or storing them.

Consent for blastocyst donation should be obtained from each donor at the time of donation. Even people who have given prior indication of their intent to donate to research any blastocysts that remain after clinical care should nonetheless give informed consent at the time of donation. Donors should be informed that they retain the right to withdraw consent until the blastocysts are actually used in cell line derivation.

The current regulatory system specifies basic elements of information that must be provided to prospective participants during the informed consent process. In the context of donation for research, disclosure should ensure that potential donors understand the risks involved, if any. Potential donors should be told of all options concerning the handling and disposition of their blastocysts, including freezing for later use, donation to others for reproductive use, research use, or disposing of them in accordance with the facility's policies and practices. To the extent possible, potential donors should be informed of the array of future research uses before giving consent to donate blastocysts for research. Comprehensive information should be provided to all donors that is readily accessible and at a level that will facilitate an informed decision. Written informed consent should be obtained from all those who elect to donate blastocysts or gametes.

Adherence to Standards of Clinical Care

Clinical facilities that provide assisted reproductive technology services are obligated to protect the rights and safety of their patients and to behave in an ethical manner. Researchers should not pressure members of the fertility treatment team to generate more oocytes than necessary for the optimal chance of reproductive success. An IVF clinic or other third party responsible for obtaining consent or collecting materials should not be able to pay for or be paid for the material it obtains, except for specifically defined cost-based reimbursements. Such restrictions on payment to those who obtain the embryos discourage the production during routine infertility procedures of excess oocytes that might later be used for research purposes.

No member of the clinical staff should be required to participate in providing donor information or securing donor consent for research use of gametes or blastocysts if he or she has a conscientious objection to hES cell research. However, that privilege should not extend to the appropriate clinical care of a donor or recipient.

> **Consenting or refusing to donate gametes or blastocysts for research should not affect or alter in any way the quality of care provided to prospective donors. That is, clinical staff must provide appropriate care to patients without prejudice regarding their decisions about disposition of their embryos.**

> **Researchers may not ask members of the infertility treatment team to generate more oocytes than necessary for the optimal chance of reproductive success. An infertility clinic or other third party responsible for obtaining consent or collecting materials should not be able to pay for or be paid for the material obtained (except for specifically defined cost-based reimbursements and payments for professional services).**

Compliance with All Relevant Regulations

If hES cell research involves transmission of personal health information about the donors, which will increasingly be the case as cell lines approach clinical application, it will be important for investigators, institutions, and IRBs to be aware of any privacy requirements that apply through the Health Insurance Portability and Accountability Act (HIPAA). Authorization should be obtained from donors for the transmission of specific health information, which should be secured to protect donor confidentiality.

> **Investigators, institutions, Institutional Review Boards, and privacy boards should ensure that authorizations are received from donors, as appropriate and required by federal human subjects protections and the Health Insurance Portability and Accountability Act, for the confidential transmission of personal health information to repositories or to investigators who are using hES cell lines derived from donated materials.**

As the level of hES cell research in the United States increases, it is essential that institutions and investigators adhere to applicable regulatory requirements and, given the increasing frequency of international collaboration in hES cell research, it will be important to monitor regulatory developments in other countries. The ESCRO committees will be charged with ensuring that U.S. investigators follow standards and procedures consistent with current regulations and with the guidelines recommended in this report.

FDA's Good Laboratory Practice regulations pertain to the management of laboratories that are developing products that might eventually be introduced into humans (for example, in a clinical trial). Those regulations do not cover basic exploratory studies conducted to determine whether a test article has any potential utility or to determine its physical or chemical characteristics, but they do encompass *in vivo* or *in vitro* experiments to determine their safety—an activity that would be characteristic of the preclinical phase of hES cell research. Failure to conform to FDA regulations, although not itself a violation of law, would render any hES cell lines less useful if they are considered for tissue transplantation or other cell-based therapies.

Investigators and institutions involved in hES cell research should conduct the research in accordance with all applicable laws and guidelines pertaining to recombinant DNA research and animal care.

hES cell research leading to potential clinical application must be in compliance with all applicable Food and Drug Administration (FDA) regulations. When FDA requires that a link be maintained to the donor source, investigators and institutions must ensure that the confidentiality of the donor is protected, that the donor understands that a link will be maintained and that, where applicable, federal human subjects protections and the Health Insurance Portability and Accountability Act or other privacy protections are followed.

Banking of hES Cell Lines

As hES cell research advances, it will be increasingly important for institutions that obtain, store, and use cell lines to have confidence in the value of stored cells, that is, confidence that they were obtained ethically and with informed consent of donors, that they are well characterized and screened for safety, and that their maintenance and storage meet the highest scientific standards.

Institutions that are banking or plan to bank hES cell lines should establish uniform guidelines to ensure that donors of material give informed consent through a process approved by an Institutional Review Board, and that meticulous records are maintained about all aspects of cell culture. Uniform tracking systems and common guidelines for distribution of cells should be established.

The full report lays out recommended standards for any facility engaged in obtaining and storing hES cell lines (see Chapter 5).

National Policy Review

As individual states and private entities move into hES cell research, it is important to initiate a national effort to provide a formal context in which the complex moral and oversight questions associated with this work can be addressed. The state of hES cell research and clinical practice and public policy surrounding these topics are in a state of flux and are likely to be so for several years. Therefore, the committee believes that some body should be established to review the policies and guidelines covering appropriate practices in this field, but not to review and approve specific research protocols, an activity that will best occur at the local institutional level. Such a body should periodically review the adequacy of the guidelines proposed in this report in light of changes in the science and emergence of new issues of public interest. New policies and standards may be appropriate for issues that cannot now be foreseen. The organization that sponsors this body should be politically independent and without conflicts of interest, should be respected in the lay and scientific communities, and able to call on suitable expertise to support this effort.

A national body should be established to assess periodically the adequacy of the guidelines proposed in this document and to provide a forum for a continuing discussion of issues involved in hES cell research.

CONCLUSION

Research using hES cells offers great promise for future improvements in health care. To realize those benefits, further research will be required, including derivation of additional hES cell lines and testing of their potential. Such research is already in progress in many institutions and there is a need for a common set of standards. The guidelines provided in this report focus on the derivation, banking, and use of hES cell lines. They provide an oversight process that will help to ensure that hES cell research is conducted in a responsible and ethically sensitive manner and in compliance with all regulatory requirements pertaining to biomedical research in general. Although the committee hesitates to recommend another bureaucratic entity to oversee biomedical research, in this case it believes the burden to be justified because of the special issues involved in hES cell research and because of the diverse entities that might have a role in the review process in a research institution.

The success of hES cell research rests with those conducting and supporting it. All scientific investigators and their institutions, regardless of their fields, bear the ultimate responsibility for ensuring that they conduct themselves in accordance with professional standards and with integrity. In particular, people whose research involves hES cells should work closely with oversight bodies, demonstrate respect for the autonomy and privacy of those who may donate gametes and embryos, and be sensitive to public concerns about research involving human embryos.

To help ensure that these guidelines are taken seriously, stakeholders in hES cell research—sponsors, funding sources, research institutions, relevant oversight committees, professional societies, and scientific journals, as well as investigators—should develop policies and practices that are consistent with the principles inherent in these guidelines. Funding agencies, professional societies, journals, and institutional review panels can provide valuable community pressure and impose appropriate sanctions to ensure compliance. For example, ESCRO committees and IRBs should require evidence of compliance when protocols are reviewed for renewal, funding agencies should assess compliance when reviewing applications for support, and journals should require that evidence of compliance accompanies publication of results.

1

Introduction

Stem cells are capable of self-renewal and also of differentiation into specialized cells. Some stem cells are more committed to a particular developmental fate than others; for example, they divide and mature into cells of a specific type or limited spectrum of types (such as heart, muscle, blood, or brain cells). Other stem cells are less committed and retain the potential to differentiate into many types of cells. It is believed that stem cells also form reservoirs of repair cells to replace cells and tissues that degenerate over the life span of the organism. The dual capacity of stem cells for self-renewal and for differentiation into particular types of cells and tissues offers great potential for regenerative medicine. The various types of stem cells differ substantially in these properties.

In 1998, scientists reported three separate sets of research findings related to the isolation and potential use of human embryonic stem cells. Two of the 1998 reports were published by independent teams of scientists that had accomplished the isolation and culture of human embryonic stem cells (hereafter referred to as hES cells) and human embryonic germ cells (hereafter referred to as hEG cells). One report described the work of James Thomson and his co-workers at the University of Wisconsin, who derived hES cells from a human blastocyst, comprising about 200 cells, donated by a couple that had received infertility treatments (Thomson et al., 1998). Their accomplishment was significant, because hES cells are considered by many to be the most fundamental and extraordinary of the stem cells; unlike the more differentiated adult stem cells or other cell types, they are pluripotent. (See the glossary for terminology used in this report.)

The second report described the successful isolation of hEG cells in the laboratory of John Gearhart and his colleagues at the Johns Hopkins University. That team derived stem cells from primordial gonadal tissue obtained from cadaveric fetal tissue (Shamblott et al., 1998). hEG cells, which originate from the primordial reproductive cells of the developing fetus, have properties similar to those of hES cells, although there has been less research into their potential.

The third report, an article in the November 12, 1998, edition of the *New York Times*, described work funded by Advanced Cell Technology of Worcester, Massachusetts. The report was not published in a scientific journal and therefore did not meet the higher standard of peer review, but the company claimed that its scientists had caused human somatic cells to revert to the primordial state by fusing them with cow eggs. From this fusion product, a small clump of cells resembling ES cells appears to have been isolated (Wade, 1998).

In addition to those research accomplishments, the cloning of Dolly the sheep in 1997 using a technique called somatic cell nuclear transfer or, more simply, nuclear transfer (NT), illustrated another means by which to generate and isolate hES cells. hES cell preparations could potentially be produced by using NT to replace the nucleus of a human oocyte, triggering development, and then isolating hES cells at the blastocyst stage. Such a procedure was recently described by a group of Korean scientists (Hwang et al., 2004). The advantage of using NT to derive hES cells is that the nuclear genomes of the resulting hES cells would be identical with those of the donors of the somatic cells. One obvious benefit is that this would avoid the problem of rejection if cells generated from the hES cells were transplanted into the donor. Whether this approach will be technically or economically feasible is unclear. A more likely benefit of the technology is that it would further facilitate a wide range of experiments to explore the underpinnings of genetic disease and possible forms of amelioration and cure, many of which would not be possible using hES cells derived from blastocysts generated by *in vitro* fertilization (IVF), whose nuclear genomes are not defined. Although the promise of such research is as yet unrealized, most researchers believe that it will be a critical source of both important knowledge and clinical resources.

It is important to note that stem cells made via NT result from an asexual process that does not involve the generation of a novel combination of genes from two "parents." In this sense, it may be more acceptable to some than the creation of blastocysts for research purposes by IVF (National Institutes of Health, Human Embryo Research Panel, 1994). Use of NT for biomedical research, as distinct from its use to create a human being, has been considered by several advisory groups to be ethically acceptable under appropriate conditions involving the proper review and conduct of the research (NBAC, 1997, 1999a; NRC, 2002). However, there is near universal agreement that the use of NT to produce a child should not now be permitted. The medical risks are unacceptable, and many people have additional objections concerning the nature of this form of human procreation. In some countries there are statutory bans on the use of NT for reproductive purposes (see Chapter 4).

Finally, promising research has been conducted with adult stem cells (Lanza et al., 2004; Wagers and Weissman, 2004). Adult stem cells can be obtained from various tissues of adults or in some cases from neonatal tissues. A well-known example of the use of adult stem cells is bone marrow transplantation. Hematopoietic (blood-forming) adult stem cells from bone marrow or from umbilical cord blood give rise to all the cells of the blood. Skin cell transplants similarly rely on the transfer of skin stem cells. In both examples, the tissue involved naturally renews itself from its pool of stem cells—a property that can be exploited for medical use. It is possible that similar approaches can be developed for other tissues (such as muscle). However, in many other tissues, natural self-renewal appears to be a slow process, and stem cells for such tissues are correspondingly harder to characterize and isolate. There is also the possibility that some tissues may not contain a distinct subpopulation of undifferentiated stem cells at all. Furthermore, the anatomic source of the cells (such as brain or heart muscle) might preclude easy or safe access.

There are important biological differences between embryonic and adult stem cells. Embryonic stem cells show a much greater capacity for self-renewal, can be cultured to generate large numbers of cells, and are pluripotent—they have the potential for differentiation into a very wide variety of cell types. In contrast, adult stem cells appear to be capable of much less proliferation and, in general, have a restricted range of developmental capacities; that is, they can differentiate into only a limited array of cells (Wagers and Weissman, 2004). Thus most experts consider "adult stem cell research" not to be an alternative to hES and hEG cell research, but rather a complementary and important line of investigation.

hES cells currently can be derived from three sources: blastocysts remaining after infertility treatments and donated for research, blastocysts generated from donated gametes (oocytes and sperm), and the products of NT. Cadaveric fetal tissue is the only source of hEG cells. hES and hEG cells offer remarkable scientific and therapeutic possibilities, involving the potential for generating more specialized cells or tissue. This could allow the generation of new cells to be used to treat injuries or diseases involving cell death or impairment, such as Parkinson's disease, diabetes, heart disease, spinal cord injury, and hematologic and many other disorders. In addition, understanding the biology of hES and hEG cells is critical for understanding the earliest stages of human development. Ethical concerns about the sources of hES and hEG cells, however, and fears that use of NT for research could lead to the use of NT to produce a child have fostered a great deal of public discussion and debate. Concern has also been expressed about whether and how to restrict the production of human/nonhuman chimeras when conducting research with hES cells. Such research could be tremendously useful in understanding the etiology and progression of human disease and in testing new drugs, and will be necessary in preclinical testing of both adult and embryonic stem cells and their derivatives. However, some are concerned that creating chimeras would violate social conventions built around the notion of species (Robert and Baylis, 2003).

THE NEED FOR GUIDELINES

Since 1998, the volume of research being conducted with hES cells has expanded, primarily with private funds because of restrictions on the use of federal funds for such research. Those restrictions are both legislative and by executive order. Federal legislation forbids the use of federal funds for any research that destroys an embryo, that is, is "nontherapeutic" for the embryo. That effectively prevents any use of federal funds to derive hES cells from blastocysts. Research with established hES cell lines is further limited by presidential policy: the policy announced by President George W. Bush in 2001 restricts federal funding of research with hES cells to use of specific federally approved cell lines already in existence before August 9, 2001. The policy states further that funding is available only for research with hES cell lines that were derived before August 9, 2001 from frozen human blastocysts that remained at infertility clinics and that were (1) generated for reproductive purposes, (2) donated with informed consent, and (3) donated with no financial inducements.[1] Laboratories or companies that provide cells that meet those conditions (originally thought to be roughly 60 cell lines, now thought to be about 22) could list the lines in the National Institutes of Health (NIH) Human Embryonic Stem Cell Registry. To do so they were required to submit a signed assurance that their hES cells met the criteria. Once the assurance was verified, the cell lines became available for use in federally funded hES cell research. The date of August 9, 2001, was set as the cutoff point to distance the federal government from any privately funded future use of embryos for hES cell research.

Not all the original hES cell lines thought to be available for federally funded research have been viable, nor do they exhibit sufficient genetic diversity for all research endeavors and possible future clinical use. Furthermore, the roughly 22 lines now available were grown on mouse-feeder cell layers. That does not necessarily render them inadequate for research pursuing human applications, but it does raise concerns about contamination. The presence of animal feeder cells increases the risk of transfer of animal viruses and other infectious agents to humans that receive the hES cells and in turn to many others. There is also the risk that hES cells grown with nonhuman animal products will have incorporated antigenic glycolipids into their cell surface. If hES cell research and therapy are to be thoroughly investigated, cell lines that are more genetically diverse and free of animal contaminants must be available. A first step in that direction was taken in February 2005 with the publication of a paper documenting the first successful growth of hES cell lines without mouse feeder cells, although contact with a growth supplement derived

---

[1]"Notice of Criteria for Federal Funding of Research on Existing Human Embryonic Stem Cells and Establishment of NIH Human Embryonic Stem Cell Registry (Nov. 7, 2001)", at http://grants.nih.gov/grants/guide/notice-files/NOT-OD-02-005.html.

from mouse cells and bovine serum means that the lines are not yet completely free of contact with nonhuman materials (Xu et al., 2005).

Despite the restricted use of federal funds for research, the derivation of new cell lines is proceeding legally in the private sector and in academic settings with private funds. Some states have banned some or all forms of this research (see Chapter 4), but other states are actively promoting hES cell research. Although general regulation of laboratory research exists, there are no established regulations that specifically address procedures for hES cell research.

Several academic research centers are conducting hES cell research in this uncertain funding and regulatory climate and would benefit greatly from a set of uniform standards for conduct. Privately funded hES cell research is subject to some regulation or other constraints, primarily through human subjects protection regulations, the limits placed on licensees by the holders of NT and hES cell patents, state laws, and self-imposed institutional guidelines at companies and universities now doing or contemplating this research. Those aiming to produce biological therapies are also subject to Food and Drug Administration (FDA) regulation (see Chapter 4).

Because of the absence of federal funding for most hES cell research being conducted today, some standard protections may be lacking, and the implementation of protections is almost certainly not uniform throughout the country. The techniques for deriving the cells have not been fully developed as standardized and readily available research tools and the development of any therapeutic applications remain some years away. Because there is substantial public support for this area of research (Nisbet, 2004), and because several states are moving toward supporting this research in the absence of federal funds, heightened oversight is essential to assure the public that such research can and will be conducted ethically.

Because of the void left by restriction of federal funding and its attendant oversight of research and because of the importance that the scientific and biomedical community attaches to pursuing potential new therapies with hES cell lines, the National Academies initiated this project to develop guidelines for hES cell research to advance the science in a responsible manner. The project follows a series of reports issued by the Academies on this and related topics.

The 2002 National Academies report *Stem Cells and the Future of Regenerative Medicine* (NRC, 2002a) called for human adult stem cell and hES cell research to move forward. It also concluded that so-called therapeutic cloning, or NT for research purposes, has a separate and important potential both for scientific research and for future medical therapies. The report argued for federal funding of research deriving and using hES cells from multiple sources, including NT, asserting that, without government funding of basic research concerning stem cells, progress toward medical therapies is likely to be hindered. It noted that public sponsorship of basic research would help to ensure that many more scientists could pursue a variety of research questions and that their results would be made widely accessible in scientific journals—two factors that speed progress substantially. Public funding also offers greater opportunities for regulatory oversight and scrutiny of research.

The committee recommended that, given the ethical dilemmas and scientific uncertainties raised by hES cell research, a national advisory body made up of leading scientists, ethicists, and other stakeholders should be established at NIH. It argued that the group could ensure that proposals for federal funding to work on hES cells were justified on scientific grounds and met federally mandated ethical guidelines. The committee noted that NIH had set up similar watchdog panels, such as the Recombinant DNA Advisory Committee (RAC), which oversees genetic engineering research on the basis of an extensive set of guidelines.

In the report, *Scientific and Medical Aspects of Human Reproductive Cloning* (NRC, 2002b), the National Academies called for a "legally enforceable ban" on human reproductive cloning owing to scientific and medical concerns. The report recommended that such a ban be revisited in 5 years. Despite several legislative attempts to ban the use of NT for reproductive purposes, no such prohibition exists in federal statute, although FDA has stated that it has the authority to prohibit the use of NT for reproductive purposes on the basis of safety concerns.[2] Moreover, although a voluntary moratorium has worked in the past to delay scientific research (such as recombinant DNA research), the committee judged that a voluntary moratorium was unlikely to work for human reproductive cloning, because reproductive technology is widely accessible in numerous private fertility clinics that are not subject to federal research regulations. In addition, when the RAC (a model of successful self-regulation leading to public policy) was established and its guidelines were put into place, the vast majority of research biologists in the United States were funded by NIH or the National Science Foundation, so the potential sanction—loss of federal grants—was a strong disincentive. That would not be the case for human reproductive cloning.

Other national panels have expressed views about the regulation of reproductive cloning and the use of NT for research into new therapies. President William J. Clinton's National Bioethics Advisory Commission (NBAC) also issued two reports on the issues. In its 1997 report *Cloning Human Beings*, issued before the isolation of hES cells, NBAC wrote that hES cells could provide critical strategies for cell-based therapies and that NT could be important in averting graft rejection in recipients of such therapy (NBAC, 1997). In its 1999 report *Ethical Issues in Human Stem Cell Research* (NBAC, 1999a), NBAC recommended that federal funds be available for the derivation *and* use of hES cells and that, for the moment, federal funding be restricted to research in which the cells were derived from blastocysts that remained after IVF or were derived from fetal tissue while research with cells derived in other ways remained legal and privately funded. The commission suggested that following this recommendation would make sufficient hES cells available for research. It also noted that the issue should be revisited if studies on those

---

[2]See FDA letter to investigators/sponsors at http://www.fda.gov/cber/ltr/aaclone.pdf.

cell lines demonstrate the need for federal funding of research with NT-derived cell lines or cell lines from blastocysts generated for research purposes.

In its 1999 report, NBAC outlined a system of national oversight to review protocols, monitor research, and ensure strict adherence to guidelines. Although intended for research with hES cells derived from IVF blastocysts, many of the recommendations could apply equally well to blastocysts derived using NT. NBAC's regulatory paradigm was based in part on the regulatory system already in place governing fetal tissue transplantation research: strict oversight and separation of the decision to terminate a pregnancy from the decision to donate material.

In its 2002 report, *Human Cloning and Human Dignity: An Ethical Inquiry,* 10 of 17 members of President Bush's Council on Bioethics recommended a 4-year moratorium on "cloning-for-biomedical-research." They also called for "a federal review of current and projected practices of human embryo research, pre-implantation genetic diagnosis, genetic modification of human embryos and gametes, and related matters, with a view to recommending and shaping ethically sound policies for the entire field." The advocates of the moratorium argued that it "would provide the time and incentive required to develop a system of national regulation that might come into use if, at the end of the four-year period, the moratorium were not reinstated or made permanent." Furthermore, they argued that "in the absence of a moratorium, few proponents of the research would have much incentive to institute an effective regulatory system."

Seven members of the 17-member council voted for "permitting cloning-for-biomedical-research now, while governing it through a prudent and sensible regulatory regime." They argued that research should be allowed to go forward only when the necessary regulatory protections to avoid abuses and misuses of cloned embryos are in place. "These regulations might touch on the secure handling of embryos, licensing and prior review of research projects, the protection of egg donors, and the provision of equal access to benefits."

Finally, in September 2003, a worldwide movement of science academies led to a major meeting in Mexico City in which 66 academies—including the U.S. National Academy of Sciences—from all parts of the world and all cultural traditions and religions called for a global ban on the use of NT for human reproduction as a matter of urgency. The group of academies specified that no ban on NT for human reproduction should preclude hES cell research with NT blastocysts. A growing number of countries have far more permissive policies regarding such research than the United States has (Walters, 2004; see also Chapter 4).

Because there is widespread agreement in the international scientific community about the potential value of hES cell research—including the use of NT to derive hES cell lines—and because there is, at present, general agreement that NT should not be used to produce a child, the best possible way to move forward with hES cell research in pursuit of new therapies is to have a set of guidelines to which the U.S. scientific community can adhere.

A key reason for the remarkable success of science since its emergence in modern form—besides the application of the scientific method itself—is the communal nature of scientific activity. The tradition of sharing materials and results with colleagues speeds scientific progress and symbolizes to the nonscientific world that in the final analysis the goal of science is to expand knowledge and improve the human condition. Not all scientists want to or have the resources to derive new stem cell lines, so the ability to share cell lines will create greater access for qualified scientists to participate in human stem cell research. A uniform set of criteria for deriving hES cell lines and reviewing research will help to assure that research institutions that derive, store, and maintain hES cells meet a standard set of requirements for provenance and ethical review.

Another positive aspect of a set of established and generally agreed upon guidelines would be greater public confidence in the conduct of hES cell research. The integrity of privately funded hES cell research would be enhanced in the public's perception as well as in actuality by the existence of a standardized set of guidelines. Public confidence would also be increased by enhanced understanding of the research. Some of the concerns about hES cell research arise from lack of familiarity with the scientific issues. It is especially crucial that the public have access to accurate information and the scientific community needs to make greater efforts to explain what research is being proposed and why. Patient advocacy groups and those with a stake in the potential therapeutic benefits of such research have begun to provide some of the education that has been lacking. As part of the larger society, the scientific community and the lay public need to engage in constructive discussion about this and other promising new fields of biomedical research to ensure that public confidence is maintained.

A BRIEF HISTORY OF U.S. DISCUSSIONS AND POLICIES REGARDING RESEARCH INVOLVING HUMAN EMBRYOS

Public debates and deliberations about embryo research have extended over the last 30 years. In 1975, the Secretary of the Department of Health, Education, and Welfare (DHEW) announced that the department would fund no proposal for research on human embryos or on IVF unless it was reviewed and approved by a federal ethics advisory board. IVF was still an experimental technique: Louise Brown, the first IVF baby, was born in 1978 in the United Kingdom. The human subjects regulations that resulted from the work of the National Commission for the Protection of Human Subjects of Biomedical and Behavioral Research (National Commission) required review of such work by an Ethics Advisory Board (EAB) to be appointed by the DHEW Secretary (National Commission, 1975). In 1977, NIH received an application from an academic researcher for support of a study involving IVF. After the application had undergone scientific review by NIH, it was forwarded to the EAB. At its May 1978 meeting, the EAB agreed to review the research proposal and later approved it for initiation.

With the increased public interest that followed the birth of Louise Brown that summer, the Secretary of DHEW asked the EAB to study the broader social, legal, and ethical issues raised by human IVF. On May 4, 1979, in its report to the Secretary, the EAB concluded that federal support for IVF research was "acceptable from an ethical standpoint," provided that some conditions were met, such as informed consent for the use of gametes, an important scientific goal that was "not reasonably attainable by other means" and not maintaining an embryo "*in vitro* beyond the stage normally associated with the completion of implantation (14 days after fertilization)" (DHEW EAB 1979, 106, 107). No action was ever taken by the Secretary with respect to the board's report; for other reasons, the department dissolved the EAB in 1980. Considerable opposition to the moral acceptability of IVF was expressed by some and contributed to paralysis regarding reconstitution of the EAB (Congregation, 1987).

Because it failed to appoint another EAB to consider additional research proposals, DHEW effectively forestalled any attempts to support IVF research with federal funds, and no experimentation involving human embryos was ever funded pursuant to the conditions set forth in the May 1979 report or through any further EAB review.

A 1988 report by the congressional Office of Technology Assessment about infertility forced a re-examination of the EAB (U.S. Congress, OTA, 1988), and a later House hearing focused on its absence. The DHEW Assistant Secretary promised to re-establish an EAB, and a new charter was published, but it was never signed after the election of President George H. W. Bush (Windom, 1988). The George H. W. Bush administration did not support re-establishing an EAB. The absence of a federal mechanism for the review of controversial research protocols continued until 1993, when the NIH Revitalization Act effectively ended the *de facto* moratorium on support of IVF and other types of research involving human embryos by nullifying the regulatory provision that mandated EAB review. In response, NIH Director Harold Varmus convened a Human Embryo Research Panel (HERP) to develop standards for determining which projects could be funded ethically and which should be considered "unacceptable for federal funding."

The HERP submitted its report to the Advisory Committee to the Director in September 1994.[3] In addition to describing areas of research that were acceptable and unacceptable for federal funding, the panel recommended that under certain conditions federal funding should be made available to make embryos specifically for research purposes. Acting on this submission, the Advisory Committee to the Director formally approved the HERP recommendations (including provision for the deliberate creation of research embryos) and transmitted them to the NIH Director on December 1, 1994. On December 2, pre-empting any NIH response, President Clinton intervened to clarify an earlier endorsement of embryo research,

---

[3]Available at http://www.bioethicsprint.bioethics.gov/reports/past_commissions/index.html.

stating that "I do not believe that Federal funds should be used to support the creation of human embryos for research purposes, and I have directed that NIH not allocate any resources for such requests" (Office of the White House Press Secretary, 1994).

The NIH Director proceeded to implement the HERP recommendations not proscribed by the President's clarification, concluding that NIH could begin to fund research activities involving "surplus" blastocysts. But before any funding decisions could be made, Congress took the opportunity afforded by the Department of Health and Human Services (DHHS) appropriations process (then under way) to stipulate that any activity involving the creation, destruction, or exposure to risk of injury or death of human embryos for research purposes may not be supported by federal funds under any circumstances. The same legislative rider has been inserted into later annual DHHS appropriating statutes, enacting identically worded provisions into law (the so-called Dickey-Wicker amendment, named after its congressional authors). Thus, to date, no federal funds have been used for research that requires the destruction of additional human embryos, whether generated originally for reproductive purposes or for research, although the current federal policy permits research on specific cell lines derived from blastocysts prior to August 2001.

When the reports of the successful isolation of hES cell lines were published in 1998, the question arose as to whether it was acceptable to provide federal funding for hES cell research that would use embryonic stem cells that were obtained from IVF blastocysts with private funding. The NIH Director sought the opinion of the DHHS General Counsel regarding the effect of the appropriations rider to the NIH Revitalization Act. The General Counsel reported that the legislation did not prevent NIH from supporting research that uses hES cells derived using private funding because the cells themselves do not meet the statutory, medical, or biological definition of a human embryo (NIH OD, 1999). Having concluded that NIH may fund both internal and external research that uses hES cells but does not create or actively destroy human embryos, NIH delayed funding until an ad hoc working group developed guidelines for the conduct of ethical research of this kind. These guidelines prescribed the documentation and assurances that had to accompany requests for NIH funding of research with human hES cells, and designated certain areas of hES cell research that were ineligible for NIH funding:

- the derivation of hES cells from human embryos,
- research in which hES cells are utilized to create or contribute to a human embryo,
- research utilizing hES cells that were derived from human embryos created for research purposes rather than for fertility treatment,
- research in which hES cells are derived using NT, that is, the transfer of a human somatic cell nucleus into a human or animal oocyte,
- research utilizing hES cells that were derived using NT,

- research in which hES cells are combined with an animal embryo, and
- research in which NT is used for the reproductive cloning of a human.

Before any grants could be funded, the 2000 election produced a new administration, and consequently the policies that exist today. As previously noted, on August 9, 2001, President Bush announced that NIH could fund research that uses hES cells but only if the cell lines had been derived prior to that date. The President maintained further that the guidelines for hES cell research developed during the Clinton presidency and the ethics advisory committee itself were no longer needed. Instead, an NIH Stem Cell Task Force composed entirely of NIH personnel was appointed to "focus solely on the science" of stem cell research. That might be explained by the fact that many of the remaining ethical guidelines that NIH had planned to put into effect were no longer needed, because they applied to issues surrounding federal funding of research on hES cell lines yet to be derived.

Meanwhile, other countries have been active in developing laws and regulations governing research in this area (see Chapter 4). In addition, in the United States a patchwork of state laws and programs ranges from a complete ban on all hES cell research to a new program recently enacted in California that funds the development of new lines derived from both IVF blastocysts and using NT.

STATEMENT OF TASK

In light of the absence of federal guidelines, the Committee on Guidelines for Human Embryonic Stem Cell Research was asked to develop voluntary guidelines to encourage responsible practices in hES cell research—regardless of source of funding—including the use and derivation of new stem cell lines derived from surplus blastocysts, from blastocysts generated with donated gametes, and through the use of NT. The guidelines should take ethical and legal concerns into account and encompass the basic science and health sciences policy issues related to the development and use of hES cells for research and eventual therapeutic purposes, such as

1. Recruitment of blastocyst, gamete, or somatic cell donors, including medical exclusion criteria, informed consent, the use of financial incentives, risks associated with egg retrieval, confidentiality, and the interpretation of genetic information developed from studies that use these materials and might have importance to the donor.
2. The characterization of stem cells for purposes of standardization and for validation of results.
3. The safe handling and storage of blastocysts and stem cell material and the conditions for transfer of such material among laboratories.

4. Prerequisites to hES cell research (such as examination of alternative approaches), appropriate uses of hES cells in research or therapy, and limitations on the use of hES cells.
5. Safeguards against misuse.

In accordance with the stated position of the National Academies that there should be a global ban on NT for human reproduction (NRC, 2002), the guidelines developed by this committee focus exclusively on research and therapeutic uses of hES cells and NT.

To conduct its work, the committee surveyed the current state of science in this field and likely pending developments, reviewed the policy and ethical issues posed by the research, examined professional and international regulations and guidelines affecting hES cell research, and conducted a 2-day workshop with speakers who represented many scientific, ethical, and public policy perspectives. It did not revisit the debate about whether hES cell research should be pursued; rather it assumed that both hES cell and adult stem cell research would continue in parallel with federal and nonfederal funding. In addition, although the committee recognizes that successful resolution of intellectual property issues will be critically important in this evolving area of research, it was beyond its charge and beyond its capabilities to address adequately all of the legal issues that will arise. Chapter 4 briefly addresses ongoing efforts to ensure that intellectual property issues do not impede new developments in biomedical research.

The guidelines presented in Chapter 6 focus on the procurement of embryos and gametes and the derivation, banking, and use of hES cell lines. They provide an oversight process that will help to ensure that research is conducted in a responsible and ethically sensitive manner and in compliance with all regulatory requirements pertaining to biomedical research in general. These guidelines are being issued for use by the scientific community, including researchers in university, industry, or other private sector research organizations, as well as practitioners of assisted reproduction, which will be one of the sources of donated embryos and gametes.

PRECEDENTS FOR SCIENTIFIC SELF-REGULATION

Perhaps the archetype of modern scientific self-regulation in the life sciences— although primarily focused initially on safety rather than ethical issues— was the moratorium on recombinant DNA research that emerged from a meeting of several hundred scientists at the Asilomar Conference Center in California. A controversy had erupted in 1971 about an experiment that involved inserting genes from a monkey virus, SV40, which can make rodent cells cancerous, into an *E. coli* bacterial cell. Prominent scientists called for a halt to recombinant DNA research until the matter could be resolved. The 1975 Asilomar conference concluded that safeguards should be introduced into recombinant DNA work, ultimately including the creation of the NIH RAC and guidelines for federally funded recombinant DNA research. It is generally agreed that the Asilomar conference and the measures that followed helped to reassure Congress and the public that the scientific community took its responsibilities seriously and allowed the research to go forward.

Although the recombinant DNA debate and its results have achieved a sort of iconic status in the annals of science's self-regulation, less spectacular examples have also arisen in the absence of or as a complement to government regulation of science and medicine. The government often relies on the private sector to regulate itself and supports it with the threat of sanctions. An example is the Joint Commission for the Accreditation of Health Care Organizations; failure to meet its standards can result in the loss of Medicare reimbursement. In the field of assisted reproduction, the lack of government funding has resulted in professional efforts to generate standards, such as those promulgated by the American Society for Reproductive Medicine (ASRM) and the Society for Assisted Reproductive Technologies.

Because there is no current federal support of hES cell research in which new cell lines are derived, the most applicable sets of guidelines in the United States for this purpose come from the Ethics Committee of the ASRM (ASRM, 2000, 2004b). Most international guidelines also call for some special oversight body for stem cell research to review documentation of compliance with the guidelines of various government agencies, both domestic and foreign. Such evaluation is in some cases folded into the evaluation of scientific merit; in others it is performed by stand-alone ethics review bodies. In the United States, review of scientific merit is typically conducted by the funding agency, which is often a federal agency. That will not be the case, for the time being, for most hES cell research conducted in this country.

There are clear advantages to government action, especially with regard to the legal standing of industry standards. Outstanding examples relevant to this report and to cultural environments that are similar to the United States are the British Human Fertilisation and Embryology Authority and the more recent Canadian Assisted Human Reproduction Agency. But in the absence of such arrangements, our proposals for a system of local review combined with a national oversight panel would go far toward consolidating and monitoring the policies and practices of hES cell research.

CONCLUSION

In the absence of federal guidelines broadly governing the generation and research use of hES cells, the scientific community and its institutions should step forward to develop and implement its own, much in the spirit of Asilomar, which resulted in the RAC guidelines in use today. Such guidelines are needed by the scientific community as a framework for hES cell research and would reassure the public and Congress that the scientific community is attentive to ethical concerns and is capable of self-regulation while moving forward with this important research. The premise is not to advocate that the work be done—that has already been debated with some consensus reached in the scientific community and elsewhere—

but rather to start with the presumption that the work is important for human welfare, that it will be done, and that it should be conducted in a framework that addresses scientific, ethical, medical, and social concerns. The public increasingly supports this area of research and its potential to advance human health.

The next chapter describes the current status of research involving hES cells. It also addresses possible novel sources of hES cell lines not yet developed and the use of human/nonhuman chimeras in research.

Chapter 3 focuses on ethical and policy issues and how existing and proposed guidelines address them. In Chapter 3, the committee proposes a local review mechanism to oversee research involving hES cells. It also recommends establishing a national body to periodically update the guidelines recommended in this report and assess the status of the field. Chapter 4 describes the current legal and regulatory environment of hES cell research in the United States and around the world. Chapter 5 addresses recruitment of donors and the informed consent process and makes recommendations about review of the processes by which donated materials are obtained. Chapter 5 also discusses the need for some standards in the banking and maintenance of hES cell lines. The final chapter consolidates the recommendations made in previous chapters as formal guidelines.

2

Scientific Background of
Human Embryonic Stem Cell Research

INTRODUCTION

Human embryonic stem cells (hES cells) are primitive (undifferentiated) cells that can self-renew or differentiate into most or all cell types found in the adult human body (Edwards, 2004; Gardner, 2004). Differentiation is the process whereby an unspecialized cell acquires specialized features, such as those of a heart, liver, or muscle cell.

Fertilization of an oocyte by a sperm results in a one-cell zygote, which begins to divide without any increase in size (Figure 2.1). By 3-4 days after fertilization, cell division results in a compact ball of 16-32 cells known as a morula. By 5-6 days, a blastocyst is formed consisting of a sphere of about 200-250 cells. The sphere is made up of an outer layer of cells (the trophectoderm), a fluid-filled cavity (the blastocoel), and a cluster of cells in the interior (the inner cell mass). Up to this point, there has been no net growth (Figure 2.1). The cells of the inner cell mass will give rise to the embryonic disk and ultimately the fetus, but not the placenta, which arises from the trophectoderm. Neither the trophectoderm nor the inner cell mass alone can give rise to a developing fetus. After the blastocyst implants into the uterus (day 6), the cells of the inner cell mass differentiate to form the embryonic tissue layers of the developing fetus. Embryonic stem cells are usually derived from the primitive (undifferentiated) cells of the inner cell mass, which have the potential to become a wide variety of specialized cell types. Because embryonic stem cells can become all cell types of the body, they are considered to be pluripotent. Study of embryonic stem cells provides information about how an organism develops from a single cell and how healthy cells can potentially replace damaged cells in adult

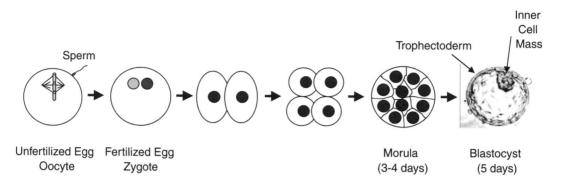

Sperm

Trophectoderm

Inner
Cell
Mass

Unfertilized Egg   Fertilized Egg
Oocyte   Zygote   Morula   Blastocyst
(3-4 days)   (5 days)

FIGURE 2.1 Preimplantation development. The oocyte (unfertilized egg) combines with sperm to form a zygote (fertilized egg). Each gamete (oocyte or sperm) is haploid (has a single set of chromosomes); the zygote and all later cells are diploid (have two sets of chromosomes). The zygote then divides approximately once a day. Since there is no growth during this period of cell division (cleavage), the cells become progressively smaller. By 3-4 days, a ball of cells (morula) has formed. By 5 days, it has become hollowed out to form a blastocyst, which consists of a sphere 0.1-0.2 mm in diameter comprising two cell types—an outer shell of trophectoderm cells and an inner collection of 30-34 cells called the inner cell mass. By day 6, the blastocyst would normally implant into the uterine wall, the trophectoderm would begin to form the placenta, and the inner cell mass would begin to form the cells and tissues of the fetus. At the blastocyst stage, cells of the inner cell mass are undifferentiated and pluripotent; that is, they have the potential to differentiate into all cells of the fetus except the placenta. If separated from the blastocyst and cultured, the cells of the inner cell mass can be converted into embryonic stem cells that are also pluripotent and can be propagated extensively while maintaining that potential. Blastocyst picture from http://stemcells.nih.gov/info/scireport/chapter3.asp.

organisms. The latter subject raises possibilities of cell-based therapies to treat disease, often referred to as regenerative medicine.

Scientists discovered how to obtain or derive embryonic stem cells from mouse blastocysts in the early 1980s (Evans and Kaufman, 1981; Martin, 1981) by culturing inner cell masses on feeder layers of mouse fibroblasts. It was later discovered that feeder cells could be replaced with culture medium containing the growth factor leukemia inhibitory factor (LIF)(Smith et al., 1988; Williams et al., 1988). Mouse ES cells (mES cells) have been studied in the laboratory, and a great deal has been learned about their essential properties and what makes them different from specialized cell types.

mES cells are shown to be pluripotent using three kinds of tests. The first and most rigorous test is to inject mES cells into the blastocoel cavity of a blastocyst (Stewart, 1993). The blastocyst is then transferred to the uterus of a pseudopregnant female (a female primed to accept implanted blastocysts). If the mES cells are pluripotent, the resulting progeny will be a chimera because it consists of a mixture of tissues and organs derived from both the donor mES cells and the recipient blastocyst. In some cases, a fetus can be derived entirely from mES cells by providing trophectoderm cells from another source (Nagy et al., 1990, 1993). However, mES cells cannot themselves form a functional placenta and therefore are not equivalent to an intact blastocyst. The ability of mES cells to generate a complete embryo tends to decline with the number of times the cells have divided (or been "passaged") in culture.

A second approach for testing pluripotency of mES cells is to inject them into the testis or under the skin or kidney capsule of an immunodeficient mouse. If pluripotent, the injected cells form benign tumors known as teratomas. The teratomas contain differentiated tissues from all three germ layers (ectoderm, mesoderm, and endoderm). Such structures as gut, muscle (smooth, skeletal, and cardiac), neural tissue, cartilage, bone, and hair are found, but they are arranged in a disorganized manner (Martin, 1981).

A third approach for testing pluripotency of mES cells is by *in vitro* differentiation (Wiles, 1993). Spontaneous differentiation can occur if the mES cells are grown in suspension without feeders or LIF. The cells will form fluid-filled clumps called embryoid bodies, which will differentiate along the ectoderm, mesoderm, and endoderm pathways. If the embryoid bodies are allowed to attach to the tissue culture dish, they will differentiate into multiple tissue types much like teratomas.

Developmentally relevant signaling factors can also be used to induce mES cells to differentiate into specific cell types *in vitro,* including hematopoietic stem cells, beating cardiac muscle cells, neuronal progenitors, endothelial cells, and bone cells. In some cases, those differentiated cell types can be transplanted into animals to form functional tissues (Lanza et al., 2004). Such work engenders excitement about regenerative medicine using hES cells. One of the milestones of mES cell research was the development of methods to modify the cells genetically (Doetschman et al., 1987; Thomas and Capecchi, 1987). The evolution of those methods has revolutionized animal models for biomedical research by allowing one to modify endogenous genes or to tag the cells so that they can be easily visualized in the animal.

Bongso et al. (1994) first described isolation and culture of cells of the inner cell mass of human blastocysts in 1994, and techniques for deriving and culturing stable hES cell lines were first reported in 1998 (Thomson et al., 1998). The trophectoderm was removed from day-5 blastocysts, and the inner cell mass, consisting of only 30-34 cells, was placed into tissue culture. Cell lines similar to mES cells were derived after fairly extensive culture and passaging of the cells. Cells with similar properties were reported at about the same time from culturing cells isolated from fetal genital ridges—so-called human embryonic germ (hEG) cells (Shamblott et al., 1998). It had previously been shown that the germ cells in fetal mouse gonads can give rise to permanent pluripotent stem cell lines in culture, mEG cells (Matsui et al., 1992; Resnick et al., 1992). Under appropriate culture conditions, hES cells were shown to be pluripotent by differentiating into multiple tissue types (Itskovitz-Eldor et al., 2000; Reubinoff et al., 2000). Since 1998, research teams have refined the techniques for growing hES cells *in vitro* (Amit et al., 2000; Itskovitz-Eldor et al., 2000; Klimanskaya and McMahon, 2004; Reubinoff et al., 2000). Collectively, the studies indicate that it is now possible to grow karyotypically normal hES cells (that is, with correct chromosome number) for more than a year in serum-free medium on mouse fibroblast feeder layers. Both XX (female) and XY (male) hES cell lines have been established. The cells express markers characteristic of pluripotent and proliferating cells. Work with hEG cells has also shown pluripotency and extended self-renewal, but more extensive work has been done with hES than with hEG cells.

There are differences between mouse and human ES cells (Pera and Trounson, 2004). For example, mES cells grow as rounded colonies with indistinct cell borders, while hES cell colonies are flatter and display more distinct cell borders. The two cell types also demonstrate differences in growth regulation. In general, both mES and hES cells require fibroblast feeder cell support. Current attempts to substitute for that support have required different approaches for the two species. The soluble growth factor, LIF, can substitute for a feeder cell layer in maintaining mES cells, but hES cells require a solid extracellular matrix (Matrigel) in place of the fibroblasts (Xu et al., 2005). Those examples of interspecies differences indicate that if one is to identify signals that cause stem cells to differentiate into specialized cells, work needs to continue with both hES and mES cells.

Embryonic stem cells have three important characteristics that distinguish them from other types of cells. First, hES cells express factors—such as Oct4, Sox2, Tert, Utf1 and Rex—that are associated with pluripotent cells (Carpenter and Bhatia, 2004). Second, they are unspecialized cells that renew themselves through many cell divisions. A starting population of stem cells that proliferates for many months in the laboratory can yield millions of cells. An important research challenge is to understand the signals that cause a stem cell population to remain unspecialized and to continue to proliferate until they are needed for repair of a specific tissue.

A third characteristic of hES cells is that under some physiological or experimental conditions in tissue culture they can be induced to become cells with special functions, such as cardiomyocytes (the beating cells of the heart), liver cells, nerve cell precursors, endothelial cells, hematopoietic cells, and insulin-secreting cells (Assady et al., 2001; Chadwick et al., 2003; Kaufman et al., 2001; Kehat et al., 2001; Levenberg et al., 2002; Mummery et al., 2002; Reubinoff et al., 2001; Reubinoff et al., 2000; Xu et al., 2002; Zhang et al., 2001). However, because hES cells have not yet been used in blastocyst chimera studies, researchers have been able to assess *in vivo* differentiation only after injection of hES cells into immunodeficient mice. There, the cells create teratomas in which tissues of the three embryonic germ layers are found (Thomson et al., 1998). Examples are bone and cartilage tissue, striated muscle, gut-like structures, neural rosettes, and glomerulus-like structures. More organized structures—such as hair follicles, salivary glands, and tooth buds—also form. hES cells will also create embryoid bodies and differentiate *in vitro* (Itskovitz-Eldor et al., 2000). However, those types of differentiation assays do not provide conclusive evidence that the resulting cell types are functioning normally, nor whether hES cells have the capacity to participate in normal development in the context of the three-dimensional embryo in the reproductive tract. Such conclusive evidence requires testing in blastocyst chimeras as is routinely done with mES cells.

Understanding why ES cells are able to proliferate essentially indefinitely and retain the ability to be induced to differentiate and stop proliferating will provide important information about the regulation of normal embryonic development and the uncontrolled cell division that can lead to cancer. It is known that external signals for cell differentiation include chemicals secreted by other cells, physical contact with neighboring cells, and molecules in the microenvironment. Identifying such factors would allow scientists to find methods for controlling stem cell differentiation in the laboratory and thereby allow growth of cells or tissues that can be used for specific purposes, such as cell-based therapies.

Several methods have been shown to be effective for delivering exogenous genes into hES cells, including transfection by chemical reagents, electroporation, and viral infection (Eiges et al., 2001; Gropp et al., 2003; Ma et al., 2003; Pfeifer et al., 2002; Zwaka and Thomson, 2003). Those are all critical methodological objectives that must be met if hES cells are to be used as the basis of therapeutic transplantation.

NUCLEAR TRANSFER TO GENERATE STEM CELLS

Most work on hES cells has taken place with a relatively small number of cell lines obtained from excess blastocysts donated from *in vitro* fertilization (IVF) programs. The genetic makeup of the cells is not controlled in any way, and genetic variation among lines needs to be considered when results from different lines are compared. Experience from research with mES cells shows that ES cell lines can differ markedly in their differentiation efficiencies. Being able to control the genotype of ES cells would be valuable for various reasons, most notably the desire to generate ES cells with genotypes known to predispose to particular diseases. In the case of single-gene defects, one could achieve that goal by deriving hES cells from discarded morulae or blastocysts that were identified with preimplantation genetic diagnosis (PGD) procedures (Verlinsky et al, 2005) as carrying mutations or by generating the appropriate mutation by gene targeting of established hES cell lines. However, such approaches cannot be used if the genetic predisposition has an unknown basis or arises from multiple gene effects. Availability of hES cell lines from patients with Alzheimer's disease, type I diabetes, or many other complex diseases would provide a source of cells that could be differentiated into appropriate cell types; and the progression of the disease could then be modeled and potentially modified in culture. Given the complex interplay between genotype and environment that typifies complex chronic diseases, the availability of cell-line models would provide major new tools for diagnosis and therapy. In this context, hES cells are research tools for the study of disease, not therapeutic agents themselves.

Controlling the genotype of ES cells will also be important in the future if they are to be used directly as therapeutic tools in regenerative medicine. Transplantation of hES cells will face issues of tissue rejection common to all forms of organ or tissue transplants. As in organ or bone marrow transplantation, one solution is to develop large banks of genetically diverse hES cells to increase the chances that matches can be found for all patients who need them. That is one strong medical reason for generating additional hES cell lines from a wider spectrum of the population. Other methods to overcome tissue rejection, including genetic modification of hES cells to reduce immunogenicity and use of immunosuppressive drugs may be helpful. However, in the long run, one obvious solution would be autologous transplantation, using hES cells genetically identical with the recipient of the graft.

Generation of ES cells using nuclear transfer (NT) has the potential to produce ES cells of defined genotype to address both genetic diversity and avoidance of rejection. NT is the process by which the DNA-containing nucleus of any specialized cell (except eggs and sperm, which contain only half the DNA present in other cells) is transferred into an oocyte whose own nuclear genome has been removed (Figure 2.2). The egg can then be activated to develop and will divide to form a blastocyst, whose genetic material and genetically determined traits are identical with those of the donor of the specialized cell, not those of the donor of the oocyte. The oocyte does provide a very small amount of genetic information in the mitochondria, the "energy factories" of the cell, but the genes in the nucleus are of overriding importance, nuclear genes being responsible for the vast majority of the traits of the animal. If such a blastocyst were transferred to a uterus, the transferred blastocyst could potentially develop into a live-born offspring—a clone of the nuclear donor. NT was first developed with frog embryos and later successfully used to generate Dolly the sheep, the first mammal cloned from an adult cell (Campbell et al., 1996). Since the birth of Dolly, live cloned offspring of several other mammalian species have been reported, including mice, goats, pigs, rats, cats, and cows. The success rate of live births is very low, however, and a variety of abnormalities have been found in cloned animals (NRC, 2002b), so this is currently an unreliable technology and unsafe for application to humans. Given the safety issues associated with NT for human reproduction, there is a worldwide consensus that such efforts should be not be conducted at this time. Despite some well-publicized but undocumented claims of production of live cloned babies, the scientific community in general and this committee in particular support that moratorium.

Blastocysts derived using NT can be an important source of genetically defined ES cells. If the inner cell mass of the NT-derived blastocyst, comprising a few dozen undifferentiated cells, is removed and grown in culture, ES cells can be derived and their genotype will be identical with that of the nuclear donor. Successful derivation of pluripotent mES cells from cloned NT blastocysts has been demonstrated in mice by several groups (Kawase et al., 2000; Munsie et al., 2000; Wakayama et al., 2001). In addition, the principle of alleviating a genetic disease was demonstrated by transplantation of genetically repaired mouse NT ES cells in an immunodeficient

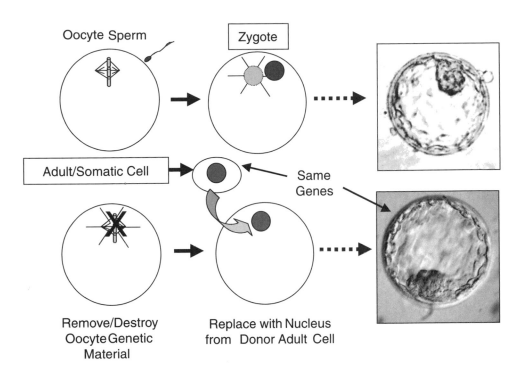

Oocyte Sperm

Zygote

Adult/Somatic Cell

Same Genes

Remove/Destroy Oocyte Genetic Material

Replace with Nucleus from Donor Adult Cell

FIGURE 2.2 Comparison of Normal Preimplantation Development with Nuclear Transfer (NT). In NT, the genetic material of the oocyte is removed and replaced with a diploid nucleus from a somatic (body) cell. This divides to yield an NT blastocyst whose genes are identical with those of the donor somatic cell. NT blastocysts, like normal blastocysts, can be used to derive embryonic stem cells from their inner cell masses. The picture shown is of a normal human blastocyst (http://www.fosep.org/images/blastocyst2.gif) because pictures of human NT blastocysts are scarce and normal and NT blastocysts appear indistinguishable.

mouse (Rideout et al., 2002). Although production of normal live offspring from NT blastocysts is not very successful in any species, NT ES cells seem to be able to differentiate normally in mice and have been able to contribute extensively to adult tissues, including the germ line, in chimeras (Wakayama et al., 2001). The rate of successful production of ES cells from NT-derived blastocysts is, however, still quite low (less than 5 percent).

In 2004, the first report of an NT-derived hES cell line was made by Woo Suk Hwang and colleagues in South Korea (Hwang et al., 2004). One line was produced by transfer of a nucleus from donated ovarian cumulus cells to an enucleated host oocyte derived from the same donor. The line appeared to be pluripotent and chromosomally normal. Successful production of hES cells was again inefficient—

over 200 oocytes were used in the course of the experiments that generated a single line. However, the scientists made a number of improvements in the procedure as the experiments progressed, increasing the yield of blastocysts and suggesting that the success rate will be improved in the future. This proof of the principles behind generating NT hES cells has made plausible the derivation of more such lines from specifically defined genetic backgrounds.

It is important to note that stem cells made using NT result from an asexual process that does not involve the generation of a novel combination of genes from two "parents." In this sense, it may be more acceptable to some than the creation of blastocysts for research purposes by IVF (NIH HERP, 1994). It has also been suggested (Hurlbut, 2004) that transfer of genetically altered nuclei incapable of directing full development might make NT acceptable. However, it has been pointed out (Melton et al., 2004) that this approach faces many technical hurdles and does not avoid the need for oocyte donation. At least three methods for generating hES cells from defective embryos have been suggested. One such method involves the use of viable blastomeres extracted from a morula or blastocyst that has been declared dead due to cleavage arrest (Landry and Zucker, 2004). This proposal is untested and is technically challenging. Even if it were possible to identify unequivocally embryos with no chance of further development, the likelihood of then isolating a viable blastomere and generating an ES line is small. There has been only one published report claiming derivation of mES cell lines from isolated 8-cell blastomeres (Delhaise et al., 1996). One cell line was obtained from 52 fully viable, dissociated 8-cell stage morulae.

Two other methods of generating hES cells from defective embryos have been considered: parthenogenesis and androgenesis. In parthenogenesis, an oocyte can be activated to develop without being fertilized by a sperm. The genomic DNA of the resulting embryo is completely maternally derived, which is not compatible with survival to term. Both mouse and nonhuman primate parthenogenetic ES cell lines have been established (Kaufman et al., 1983; Cibelli et al., 2002). The results are of interest because deriving stem cells from parthenogenetic blastocysts could eliminate the requirement to produce and destroy viable blastocysts. Parthenogenetic ES cells could serve as an alternative source for autologous cell therapy. However, parthenogenetic mES cells show restricted tissue contributions in chimeras and in teratomas formed by grafting the cells under the kidney capsule (Allen et al., 1994); this is related to the lack of expression of key imprinted genes that are normally expressed from the paternal genome. In contrast with parthenogenesis, in androgenesis the entire genome comes from the male parent. Such embryos also do not survive to term. Diploid androgenetic mES cells have been derived (Mann et al., 1990), but many androgenetic ES cell chimeras died at early postnatal stages, and the ones that survived developed skeletal abnormalities. Again, the imprinting status of the cells differed from that of wild-type ES cells (Szabo et al, 1994). Thus, although the results show that androgenetic and parthenogenetic ES cells have broad developmental potential, their imprinted gene expression status is likely to restrict their therapeutic applications. Moreover, no human parthenogenetic or androgenetic stem cell lines have been established, and more research is needed to determine whether these techniques can be applied to human oocytes for production of stem cell lines.

SOURCES OF OOCYTES FOR NT ES CELLS

At current rates of success of generation of NT blastocysts and ES cells, one major limitation of expansion of this approach will be the availability of oocytes for NT. Current and possible future sources of such oocytes include excess oocytes and unfertilized oocytes from IVF procedures, oocytes matured from ovariectomies or fetal ovaries from pregnancy terminations, oocyte donation, derivation of oocytes from nonreproductive material, and use of nonhuman oocytes.

- **Excess oocytes and unfertilized eggs from IVF procedures.** During IVF, hormonal induction is used to generate oocytes for fertilization *in vitro*. Often, more oocytes are generated than are needed for reproductive purposes, and some oocytes may be available for research donation. In addition, after IVF, not all oocytes are successfully fertilized, and unfertilized oocytes would otherwise be discarded if not donated for research. Experiments to explore use of such oocytes for NT derivation of hES cells have been approved and initiated in the United Kingdom. However, this source of oocytes is limited, and the unfertilized oocytes may be of lower quality for cell line production. It is ethically problematic to consider alteration of the IVF clinical procedure to deliberately induce more oocytes than needed for reproduction, even with the consent of the participants. Thus, this source of oocytes is likely to be limited and unreliable for any major NT ES cell program.
- **Oocytes matured from ovariectomies or fetal ovaries from pregnancy terminations.** Adult as well as fetal ovaries contain a large supply of immature oocytes, which in principle could be harvested from adult ovaries donated after removal for clinical reasons or from fetal ovaries that are obtained from legal pregnancy terminations. In the case of other mammals, it is possible to mature such oocytes in culture and achieve fertilization and normal development, although the process is not efficient (O'Brien et al., 2003). In humans, success has been limited and requires an intermediate xenograft (transplantation into an animal) of the ovarian tissue for oocyte maturation. Research on how to expand the supply and how to mature human oocytes *in vitro* could make this a reasonable source of donated material.
- **Oocyte donation.** The most reliable source of oocytes for NT ES cells today seems to be direct donation of oocytes by female donors after hormonal induction and oocyte recovery. Such third-party donation has much in common with organ donation and already occurs in some IVF programs for

reproductive purposes. However, this option raises significant issues about the risks to the donors, about a possible profit motive if excessive payment is made for donated oocytes, and about the nature of informed consent in such circumstances. Altruistic donation of oocytes by family members for generation of disease-related NT ES cells might be a good alternative source of material.

- **Derivation of oocytes from nonreproductive material.** The problems of the limited pool of oocytes for NT would be alleviated if a renewable source of oocytes can be found. The recent report that cells resembling oocytes could be formed from mouse ES cells in culture (Hubner et al., 2003) is intriguing in this regard. If confirmed and extended to human ES cells, this approach could eventually provide an extensive source of oocytes or something resembling oocytes for NT.
- **Use of nonhuman oocytes.** Obtaining large numbers of oocytes from nonhuman mammals is relatively easy, and the use of such oocytes to derive NT blastocysts and stem cells has been considered. If this were successful, the nuclear genome would be entirely human, but there could be some persistence of nonhuman mitochondria in the cells. The relevance of such interspecies mixing for the growth, potential, and safety of such cells would need to be evaluated. There has been one report of putative ES cell lines produced after transfer of human nuclei to rabbit oocytes (Chen et al., 2003), but the finding needs to be confirmed and extended before this approach can be considered feasible.

Given the strong scientific rationale for generating human NT ES cells, there is an urgent need to develop new ethically acceptable sources of cytoplasmic material for reprogramming adult nuclei. Further research into the molecular mechanisms by which the oocyte cytoplasm reprograms the adult nucleus for pluripotency should lead to methods to bypass altogether the need for oocytes to achieve NT reprogramming. In the long run, it may be possible to reprogram adult cells or nuclei directly—not by transfer into oocytes but by other means, such as fusion with pluripotent ES cells or exposure to factors from such pluripotent cells.

INTERSPECIES MIXING

Interspecies mixing happens in nature, and deliberate human-made examples, such as mules, raise no ethical concerns. However, when one of the species involved is human, there is a clear need to consider ethical issues. Hybrids, such as mules, are animals derived from interbreeding between two different species. In the case of a mule, chromosomes from a horse and a donkey are brought together through the fusion of horse and donkey gametes in fertilization to produce an animal whose every cell contains genes from both parental species. Interspecies hybrids are rarely viable and no one proposes to generate interspecies hybrids involving human gametes, even if it were possible. However, there are valid scientific reasons for creating a second sort of interspecies mix in the context of hES cell research—a chimera. Chimeras, unlike genetic hybrids, consist of mixtures of cells (or, in some cases, tissues) from two different kinds of animals. Unlike the situation in hybrids, there is no commingling of genetic material in individual cells of a chimera.

Chimeras are widely used in research and medicine—xenotransplants of, for example, human skin onto mice, of human tumors into mice, and of human bone marrow into mice are already subject to regulation (for example, use of human material is regulated by Institutional Review Boards (IRBs) and animal care issues are regulated by Institutional Animal Care and Use Committees (IACUCs)). Thus, there seem to be no new ethical or regulatory issues regarding chimeras themselves. Nonetheless, because of the pluripotency of hES cells, the extent of their contributions to interspecies chimeras is uncertain, and both the need for and value of chimera experiments involving hES cells and related ethical concerns need to be considered (see Chapter 3). In stem cell research, the possible utility of interspecies mixing arises in several contexts.

Incorporation of hES Cells or Cells Derived from Them into Postnatal Animals of Another Species

Such experiments will be essential to test the potential of hES cells or their derivatives to differentiate into the desired cells and tissues and to ensure that hES cells or their derivatives do not give rise to inappropriate cell types or to tumors or have any other deleterious consequences. Such "preclinical testing" is analogous to the standard testing of drugs, transplants, and medical devices in animals before human clinical trials. It will inevitably be required by the Food and Drug Administration (FDA) en route to any application of hES cells or their derivatives or, indeed, of adult stem cells in therapeutic applications. As mentioned above, many experiments of this type have been done before and are well covered by existing regulations concerning use of human tissues and animals. The use of pig heart valves in humans is an example of routine clinical use of interspecies chimeras. The issues that are particular to hES cells concern the possibility that such cells, because of their pluripotency, could give rise to cells of the germline or the brain. That would be of less or no concern in the case of hES cell derivatives that had differentiated down particular developmental paths, for example, into cells able to make cartilage, bone, skin, or blood. But it needs consideration when pluripotent hES cells or their neural derivatives, such as neural stem cells, are used.

It seems highly unlikely that hES cells could contribute to the germline after implantation into a postnatal animal because the germline is set aside very early in fetal development. Nonetheless, the possibility could readily be addressed by ensuring that animals receiving hES cell transplants do not breed. The possibility of contribution to the brain is harder to evaluate. One purpose of introducing hES cells or human neural progenitor cells is to have them contribute to repair or regenerative processes and to yield neurons. Production of motor neurons, sensory neurons, or neurons that secrete mediators, such as dopamine, might all contribute to combating spinal-cord injuries and neurodegenerative diseases. However, the idea that human neuronal cells might participate in "higher-order" brain functions in a non-human animal, however unlikely that may be, raises concerns that need to be considered. Indeed, if such cells are to be used in human therapeutic interventions, one needs to know whether they could participate in that way in the context of a treatment. Thus, there are good reasons to explore this sort of issue through animal experiments. Studies on the brain are proceeding rapidly, but there is clearly a need for more investigation, and hES cell research in this field should proceed with due care (see Chapter 3).

Incorporation of hES Cells or Cells Derived from Them into Postgastrulation Stages of Another Species

Such experiments would allow a greater opportunity for hES cells to be properly incorporated into appropriately organized tissues and would therefore offer greater opportunities to reveal the potential of such cells. Similar experiments have been invaluable in testing the capacity of neuronal progenitors derived *in vitro* from mES cells by transplantation into chicken embryos (Wichterle et al., 2002); it seems clear that there will be a need or desire to conduct similar experiments to test the potential of hES cells and their derivatives. Indeed, preliminary experiments showing that hES cells can survive and differentiate after transplantation into chicken embryos have been reported (Goldstein et al., 2002). As noted at the outset, there seems little ethical concern about many such experiments, which resemble research approaches that have been used often in the past. For example, human hematopoietic stem cell transplantation would be equivalent to current human-to-mouse bone marrow transplantation and the same could be said for many other tissues. The sensitivities, again, arise concerning neuronal and germline cells and are perhaps more of a concern than in the case of transplantation into a postnatal animal, because the hES cells might be expected to have greater opportunity to participate. As above, the issue of germline contribution could be addressed by preventing any such chimeras from breeding. The potential for incorporation into brain functions needs research and monitoring as mentioned above.

Incorporation of hES Cells into Nonhuman Blastocysts

This approach is an obvious extension of techniques widely used in research with mES cells—namely, aggregation of morulae from two mice or injection of mES cells into mouse blastocysts. In both cases, the cells can contribute extensively to any mouse that arises from implantation of such a chimeric blastocyst. Clearly, an animal (e.g., mouse) blastocyst into which human cells are transplanted raises other issues because potentially the inner cell mass, the progenitor of the fetus, would consist of a mixture of human and mouse cells. It is not now possible to predict the extent of human contribution to such chimeras. If the recipient blastocyst were from an animal that is evolutionarily closer to a human, the potential for human contributions would appear to be greater. For these reasons, research that involves the production of such chimeras should be performed first using nonhuman primate ES cells in mouse blastocysts before proceeding to use of hES cells. The need for the use of blastocysts from larger mammals would need to be very clearly justified and nonhuman primate blastocysts should not be used at this time. Any chimeric experiments using hES cells should be subject to careful review by the institutional oversight committees described in Chapter 3. (Also see Chapter 3 for additional discussion of the ethical concerns surrounding chimeras.)

Use of Nonhuman Oocytes as Recipients of Human Somatic Nuclei in NT with the Aim of Generating hES Cell Lines Without the Need for Human Oocytes

The possibility of using nonhuman oocytes as recipients for NT was mentioned above. The procedure is not in wide use, and it is not clear how useful it will be, but it might constitute a solution to the problem of limited supplies of human oocytes. More immediately, interspecies combinations (human nucleus into nonhuman oocytes) are potentially valuable research tools that could be used to learn about reprogramming of somatic nuclei, which could be one long-term solution to the problems of tissue rejection and limited supplies of human oocytes. Such an interspecies construct would be similar to the product of human NT and would be subject to similar guidelines regarding implantation or culture beyond 14 days (the primitive streak stage) while still permitting the recovery of ES cells.

PRIORITIES FOR hES CELL RESEARCH

Although the potential for future therapeutic use of hES cells seems clear, many technical issues remain to be solved before the potential can be realized. More than a decade of research with mES cells has amply demonstrated their potential to differentiate into all cells of the body. Nonetheless, there is only limited understanding of how to direct their differentiation into well-defined paths, as would be necessary if hES cells are to be used to generate cells of specific developmental potential for therapeutic purposes. A clear example of how such research must proceed is offered by a study in which mES cells were coaxed to develop *in vitro* into precursors of motor neurons (restricted potential neuronal progenitors or neuronal stem cells), which were then transplanted into chicken embryos, where they differentiated into motor neurons (Wichterle et al, 2002). ES-cell-derived hematopoietic cells can also be used to achieve long-term hematopoietic reconstitution (Kyba et al., 2002), and cardiomyocytes from mouse ES cells have achieved reintegration into cardiac muscle (Klug et al., 1996). Much more of this type of differentiation and transplantation research will need to be done if hES cells are to be used in regenerative medicine, and much research is needed into the various steps of such protocols.

Experimental manipulations that will need to be developed with hES cells to achieve successful applications in human medicine are described below in sequence from hES cell derivation and culture, through preclinical testing and other research uses to illustrate the spectrum of hES cell research that will be necessary in the coming years and to point out the biomedical rationales for the experiments. These are the types of essential experiments for which the guidelines proposed later in this report are designed to provide a framework for ethical and responsible conduct.

- Additional hES cell lines must be generated because experience from studies of mES cells shows that lines differ in their potential and do not always retain their potential on extended culture. Furthermore, the hES cells now available do not have adequate genetic diversity.

- hES cells of defined genetic backgrounds need to be generated. In the future, such cells could be used in autologous cellular therapy, which would avoid problems of immune rejection, but that prospect is some years away. In the immediate term, hES cells with genotypes known to predispose to particular diseases would be invaluable for research into the bases of the diseases in question and for developing tests for diagnostic and therapeutic approaches (for example, drug testing). Few such genetically defined hES cells now exist, but several sources are possible. Excess blastocysts will necessarily be produced in the course of IVF and PGD procedures designed to derive blastocysts that lack disease-promoting genotypes. Excess blastocysts that are genotypically unsuitable for reproduction would normally be discarded but instead they can be used to generate hES cells (Verlinsky et al., 2005). Such blastocysts could also be generated with IVF procedures specifically for that purpose; families with genetic predispositions might well be motivated to contribute gametes altruistically. Alternatively, hES cells of the desired genotype could be generated using NT; again, altruistic donation of oocytes and nuclei would be a suitable route.

- Genetic manipulation of hES cells is another route to the generation of hES cells with defined genetic defects where the diseases are well enough understood for the relevant genes to be known. Research with such procedures would also lay the groundwork for future manipulations, such as gene therapy, to generate autologous cells in which genetic defects have been "fixed." Such *in vitro* manipulations could eventually allow gene modifications to be controlled with precision to avoid deleterious side effects. hES cells can be genetically modified by introduction of transgenes with a variety of approaches, and homologous recombination to alter the endogenous genes of the cells is also possible (Zwaka and Thomson, 2003). Further research into genetic modification of hES cells is important.

- As discussed in the section on NT, a major current limitation of widespread use of NT is the restricted availability of human oocytes, and research into the many different possibilities for alternative sources is needed. The possibilities include the maturation of immature oocytes derived from therapeutic ovariectomies or from fetal ovaries and, perhaps, of unfertilized oocytes from IVF clinics. However, a better long-term solution of the problem would be development of methods for producing renewable sources of oocytes, such as differentiation of hES cells. Studies on the latter possibility would be invaluable.

- Nonhuman oocytes might also be used for NT, and this needs further research.

- A means of reprogramming the nuclei of somatic cells, either by culturing cells under different growth conditions or by exposing the nuclei to factors from oocyte or hES cell cytoplasm, is essential. Research on the nature of epigenetic modification and means of modifying it so that somatic cell nuclei could be reprogrammed to a state equivalent to that of ES cells would make oocytes and embryos unnecessary for generating hES cells. Success in this effort would be a major advance and, therefore, while not imminent, seems a high priority for research.

- Research is needed to understand how to maintain the self-renewing capacity of hES cells over long-term culture and expansion. In the mouse, the LIF-JAK-STAT pathway of signaling molecules is necessary and sufficient for self-renewal, but it is not sufficient to maintain hES cells in the stem cell state (Daheron et al., 2004). For therapeutic applications, it will be essential to be able to propagate and expand hES cells.

- It will also be necessary to develop culture conditions that do not include mouse feeder cells and bovine serum as in most current research. Animal products will introduce complications in any future therapeutic use of hES cells, both with respect to FDA requirements and because nonhuman materials can contribute biochemical precursors to the hES cells that render them immunogenic and therefore unsuitable for transplantation (Martin et al., 2005). Initial success has been reported in replacing mouse feeder layers (Xu et al., 2005) but additional improvements in culture conditions will need to be developed and tested.

- Detailed investigation will be needed to determine the best means of ensuring stability of genotype, epigenetic status, and phenotypic properties of ES cells grown in long-term cultures for use in human therapies.

- Research is needed to determine how to direct the development of hES cells down particular pathways to generate cells restricted to specific developmental fates. It will involve exploration of different culture conditions and investigation of growth and differentiation factors that promote specified developmental fates. Such investigations will rely on ongoing research into the developmental biology of other species but will require direct studies of hES cells because there will be differences between ES cells of different species. Studies of nonhuman ES cell models and of hES cells must proceed in parallel.

- A related challenge will be the development of methods to separate progenitors of restricted developmental potential from hES cells (or methods to ensure complete conversion of hES cells into the desired cellular derivatives). mES cells transplanted to ectopic sites can generate benign tumors and such an outcome clearly would be undesirable in any cellular therapy. One can imagine methods for separating or removing persisting hES cells (such as sorting of undifferentiated cells or inducible suicide of inappropriate cells), but research will be required to ensure that such methods are effective.

- All the foregoing procedures will necessitate means of testing the potential of the derived cells to contribute usefully when implanted and for adverse side effects; such tests will undoubtedly be required by FDA before any therapeutic use. That requirement will necessitate development of protocols for effective and ethical testing of the potential of hES cells and their derivatives (or adult stem cells). Many tests can be conducted *in vitro* but *in vivo* tests will also be mandatory. As discussed above, some such tests present no particular ethical problems, and the technical issues can be addressed with further experimentation. However, some chimera experiments that can be easily envisaged raise issues pertaining to the possibilities of hES cell contributions to the brain or the germline. Research is needed to determine the likelihood of those potential concerns. It has been argued that their potential may be quite limited but a main purpose of developing hES cell-based therapies is to promote some participation of the implanted cells. Research will be necessary to discover the extent to which this is possible both to exploit the therapeutic potential and to avoid undesired contributions.

- One issue arising in any cell or tissue transplantation is immune rejection due to histocompatibility antigenic differences between people. This problem is confronted every day in organ transplantation and has been addressed with tissue-matching and immune suppression. Nevertheless it remains a problem and will affect any stem cell-based therapies (adult or embryonic) unless means can be found to avoid it. One such means is the use of autologous hES cells derived using a patient's own nuclei to generate genetically identical hES cells through NT. That approach is feasible and likely to be exploited, but it will face hurdles, such as oocyte availability, if it is to be widely used. The more genetically diverse hES cells there are available, the more likely that a histocompatible matching line can be found. That is a strong argument for development of stem cell banks (see Chapter 5). In parallel, research into ways of avoiding immune rejection should be encouraged both for standard organ transplantation and for future hES cell therapies. With ES cells and their derivatives, it may be possible to devise means of suppressing histocompatibility antigens, which clearly is not feasible with organ transplants.

- In addition to therapeutic transplantation, hES cells are good candidates for testing of therapeutic drugs. If hES cells can be directed to differentiate into specific cell types, they may be more likely to mimic the *in vivo* response of cells and tissues to the drug being tested and so offer safer models for drug screening. Similarly, hES cells could be used to screen potential toxins. Toxic agents often have different effects on different animal species and cell types, and this makes it critical to have the best possible *in vitro* models for evaluating their effects on human cells. However, it remains to be determined which differentiation stages of hES-derived cells are optimal for such practical applications. For example, what differentiation stages of ES-derived cells would be best for screening drugs or toxins or for delivering potentially therapeutic drugs?

CONCLUSION

The list of hES cell research priorities underlines the need for a broadly accepted set of guidelines to assist researchers and regulators in their design of investigations, whether funded by federal, state, philanthropic, or industrial sources. The research has great promise, but much further investigation is needed to realize the potential, and the sensitivities surrounding research with hES cells require continuing attention to the ethical and public policy issues. The next chapter discusses many of the ethical concerns raised by this research and proposes a system of oversight to address ethical and public concerns.

3

Addressing Ethical and Scientific Concerns Through Oversight

The promise of human embryonic stem (hES) cell research as described in Chapter 2 raises ethical concerns that require a public policy response. This chapter addresses the primary ethical concerns, specifically public sensitivities regarding the status of the human embryo, the need to respect those who donate gametes and embryos to research, the mixing of human and nonhuman cells, and the consensus that nuclear transfer (NT) should not be used for reproductive purposes at the present time. Those concerns and the need for uniform practices and standards in the scientific and medical communities, call for an appropriate and calibrated system of oversight. Several countries have already established laws and guidance in this field and some are described in this chapter (additional discussion can be found in Chapter 4). As discussed in Chapter 1, there is a precedent for self-regulation by the scientific community and research institutions in recombinant DNA research. The initiative taken by the scientific community in the 1970s with regard to recombinant DNA research serves as a model for self-governance in hES cell research in the absence of involvement of the federal government. In this chapter the committee recommends a system of local and national oversight of hES cell research. Because in the final analysis the issues involved are scientific and moral rather than financial the proposed oversight system should apply to all hES cell research regardless of the source of funding.

ETHICAL CONCERNS

The principle ethical and religious objection to hES cell research is that the derivation of hES cells involves the destruction of the blastocyst, which is regarded by some people as a human being. A second objection, which relates to blastocysts created for research purposes—whether through fertilization or NT—is that it is wrong to create a blastocyst with the intention of destroying it. A third objection is that some of the research depends on donor oocytes, which could result in the exploitation of women. In addition, some people are concerned about the mixing of human and nonhuman cells for research purposes. Finally, some object to the use of NT to derive hES cells because they fear that the use of NT for research purposes could lead to its use to produce a child.

The Special Status of the Human Embryo

Like all scientific work involving human embryos, hES cell research raises profound questions about the status of the human embryo, the extent to which it is justifiable to use human embryos to expand knowledge and ameliorate human suffering, and the conditions under which these goals may be pursued. Throughout its deliberations the committee was keenly aware that some view human embryos as morally equivalent to born human persons. This position takes several forms. Some argue that the identity of a future born person is present in the embryo. Others identify the moral equivalence of the human embryo to the born human person with the embryo's potentiality. Still others claim that human dignity is undermined by excessive manipulation of the human embryo regardless of the purpose and that this could lead to the abuse and exploitation of human persons more generally.

Yet even in our own society, where many hold this view in a philosophical sense, it has not been adopted as a matter of cultural practice. For example, the natural loss of an embryo in normal human reproduction is not recognized as a death that requires a funeral, and the disposal of human embryos after completion of infertility treatments is not treated as murder by the legal system. Nonetheless, in the United States in particular, hES cell research is eligible for limited federal funding because the current administration wishes to acknowledge the view of some that the destruction of embryos required to obtain new cell lines gives such lines a moral taint.

In contrast, many religious traditions—Islam, Judaism, and numerous Protestant denominations—do not recognize the human embryo before 40 days after conception as an entity that should be accorded the same moral status as a person. Among some of these traditions, there is also a strong commitment that faith must be manifest in good works and that the world itself and the persons within it should be objects of strenuous efforts to heal (National Bioethics Advisory Commission (NBAC), 1999b). To be sure, in these traditions the human embryo may have greater moral status than other collections of cells, but not so much that its cells may not be respectfully applied toward the other goals to which the faithful are committed.

There is a more general debate about the meaning of human dignity. For some, the use or creation of human embryos in research, or even the very prospect of advances in genetics and molecular biology, represent manipulations of life that undermine human dignity. In contrast, others view the effort to heal the sick as a profound moral obligation and the restoration of health and natural functions as the promotion of human dignity. In the latter view, the undifferentiated blastocyst cells that yield hES cells are a resource that should not be squandered.

This diversity of deeply held views must be respected. However, that respect does not require that we, as a society, prohibit hES cell research, but rather that our society create institutions for the oversight of this research that, with due moral seriousness, take into account the special status of the human embryo.

Respect for Donors of Human Embryos and Gametes

Like other modern technologies associated with human reproductive capacities, hES cell research often involves donated embryos or oocytes. There is a set of minimal conditions that applies to the process of obtaining embryos and gametes for research purposes, normally from *in vitro* fertilization clinics. Those conditions are reflected in policies, guidelines, and practices in the United States and elsewhere. They include restrictions on monetary and other inducements, separation between clinical decisions and decisions to donate, and the requirement of voluntary informed consent of donors through a process that has been approved by an Institutional Review Board (IRB), as specified in federal regulations for the protection of human subjects in research (45 CFR 46.107; see Chapter 4 for further discussion). A measure of respect for donors is the assurance that research using donated materials is limited to qualified investigators and that studies have scientific merit. Those issues are discussed in greater depth below and in Chapter 5.

Transferring hES Cells into Nonhuman Animals

The transfer of hES cells into nonhuman animals has received less attention than some of the other ethical and policy issues surrounding stem cell research. The transfer of human stem cells (whether adult or embryonic) or their derivatives into nonhuman animals, creating chimeric entities, will be an important laboratory technique in research with both adult and human embryonic stem cells and may have clinical applications as well. As discussed in Chapter 2, research purposes could include understanding the mechanisms by which transplanted cells localize and differentiate in a host and using the cells in preclinical testing. Human cells also could someday be grown into functioning tissues or organs in an animal for later transfer into a patient.

A different perception of the unnaturalness of mixing tissues from different sources is the idea that there are fixed species. However, the popular notion that there are clear and distinct lines between species is a notoriously unreliable categorical scheme. Taxonomies developed since Aristotle do not necessarily countenance the idea of natural kinds, and modern scientists differ in their precise definitions of interspecies boundaries. There is general agreement in the scientific community that these boundaries are to some extent arbitrary. As discussed in Chapter 2, some chimeras are viewed with equanimity (for example, pig heart valve transplants into humans), and one must be careful to distinguish legitimate concerns from discomfort arising from unfamiliarity. Although moral intuitions about the creation of chimeras may vary, it is a subject of deep moral concern to many thoughtful people for whom the creation of animals with certain kinds or quantities of human tissues, such as neural or germline cells, would be offensive. Accordingly, such research requires careful consideration and review.

Among the issues to be considered in the review of such proposals will be the number of hES cells to be transferred, what areas of the animal body would be involved, and whether the cells might migrate through the animal's body. The hES cells may affect some animal organs rather than others, raising questions about the number of organs affected, how the animal's functioning would be affected, and whether some valued human characteristics might be exhibited in the animal, including physical appearance.

Perhaps no organ that could be exposed to hES cells raises more sensitive questions than the animal brain, whose biochemistry or architecture might be affected by the presence of human cells. Human diseases, such as Parkinson's disease, might be amenable to stem cell therapy, and it is conceivable, although unlikely, that an animal's cognitive abilities could also be affected by such therapy. Similarly, care must be taken lest hES cells alter the animal's germline. Protocols should be reviewed to ensure that they take into account those sorts of possibilities and that they include ethically sensitive plans to manage them if they arise.

Various precautions seem reasonable in studies that involve the transfer of hES cells into nonhuman animals and should be considered in any prior review of a protocol. Questions that should be raised in this context include the following

- Are hES cells required, or can cells from other primates or animals be used?
- Has sufficient animal work preceded the proposed work involving hES cells?
- Might the cell transfer result in the animal's acquiring characteristics that are valued as distinctly human?
- If hES cells are to be transferred into an animal embryo or fetus, have studies (for example, with ES cells from other species or interspecies chimeras) suggested that the resulting creature would exhibit human characteristics that would be ethically unacceptable to find in an animal?
- If visible human-like characteristics might arise, have all those involved in these experiments, including animal care staff, been informed and educated about this?

Furthermore, donors of gametes and embryos should be informed that some of the hES cells derived from their donated cells and tissues might be transferred into nonhuman animals in the course of developing and testing their therapeutic potential (see Chapter 5).

Objections to the Use of NT for Reproductive Purposes

The ethical concerns about attempts to use NT to create children are well known. They include risks to the mother and the fetus that have been described in numerous reports by other advisory bodies and institutions (NBAC, 1997; NRC, 2002; President's Council on Bioethics, 2002). As discussed in Chapter 1, this is a matter on which the U.S. National Academies and the scientific community world-wide have spoken with virtually a single voice. Attempts to create a child by means of NT are ethically objectionable at this time because, on the basis of experience with other mammalian species, producing one child might require hundreds of pregnancies and many abnormal late-term fetuses could be produced. Furthermore, some authorities believe that there can never be a fully normal product of NT because of the differences in imprinting between the genes in a transplanted somatic nucleus and those in the oocyte nucleus that it has replaced (Jaenisch, 2004), as well as a failure of epigenetic reprogramming in general. Such concerns led to Food and Drug Administration efforts to prohibit NT for reproductive purposes.[1]

Even in the absence of moral justification for attempting NT for reproductive purposes, some groups have announced their intention to pursue that objective, even if merely to generate publicity. An oversight system for hES cell research that might include NT as a source of cell lines will reinforce the ethical and scientific consensus that NT for reproductive purposes has no place in legitimate research. The danger that the efforts will continue is far greater in the absence of systematic oversight with its attendant accountability and transparency.

THE NEED FOR AN OVERSIGHT SYSTEM

As a starting point for its deliberations, the Committee on Guidelines for Human Embryonic Stem Cell Research examined numerous other guidelines and regulations in use now or in the past to identify best practices and common features. Surveys of guidelines and regulations for embryo and/or hES cell research by this committee and others (Walters, 2004) revealed that common features of most, if not all, programs throughout the world include

- A prohibition on nuclear transfer for reproductive purposes.
- A prohibition on the culture of human embryos beyond 14 days after fertilization or when the primitive streak has appeared, whichever occurs first.

Most existing regulations and guidelines embody broad guiding principles. For example, most require that hES cell research projects aim to advance scientific and medical knowledge to benefit human health. Alternative methods (such as the use of existing hES cell lines or adult stem cells) must have been examined and shown to be

---

[1]See FDA letter to investigators and sponsors at http://www.fda.gov/cber/ltr/aaclone.pdf.

insufficient for projects that propose to derive new hES cell lines. And research must conform to the highest ethical and scientific standards and be conducted sensitively and in accordance with all regulatory requirements of the nation or state. For example, even under its relatively liberal policy, the United Kingdom, in its *Code of Practice for the Use of Human Stem Cell Lines*, requires that all hES cell research be conducted under special licenses obtained from the government. The rationale is, in part, to ensure protection of the status of the human embryo:

> The special regulations which govern the creation and use of human embryonic stem cells reflect the fact that the human embryo has a special moral status. The position taken by many (perhaps most) is that the embryo, unlike an infant, does not have the full rights of a person; however, its human potential gives it an intrinsic value which implies that neither its creation nor its destruction are to be treated casually, as reflected in law. A research license will not be granted unless the HFEA [Human Fertilisation and Embryology Authority] is satisfied that any proposed use of the embryos is necessary for the research and that the research is necessary or desirable for the purposes specified in the 1990 HFE Act and the 2001 Regulations. . . . Although the use of embryos for these purposes is now permitted under the law, researchers in this field should be sensitive to the fact that some people believe this practice to be morally unacceptable [MRC, 2004].

Many other sets of guidelines also contain provisions to ensure voluntary embryo donation—with a requirement of informed consent—and requirements that the confidentiality of donors be protected. Because there is no federal support in the United States for hES cell research in which new cell lines are derived, the most applicable guidelines come from the Ethics Committee of the American Society for Reproductive Medicine (ASRM, 2000; 2004b). Canada and the United Kingdom also have substantive procedural requirements regarding the recruitment of donors and informed consent. (Those and other approaches are addressed in detail in Chapter 5.) Most guidelines also call for some special oversight body for hES cell research to review documentation of compliance with the guidelines of various government agencies, both domestic and foreign (see Chapters 4 and 5). Oversight is in some cases folded into the evaluation of scientific merit; in others, it is performed by stand-alone ethics review bodies. Finally, most forms of laboratory and clinical research in the United States are subject to substantial local regulation, including provision of protections for human subjects in research, protections for laboratory animals, and the many considerations that must be addressed for research and testing of new drugs and medical devices. (The applicability of those regulatory systems to hES cell research is addressed in Chapter 4.)

In considering the ethical and policy issues that arise in connection with hES cell research, the committee subscribes to the consensus of many bioethics bodies throughout the world that a system of oversight of hES cell research should be in place. Examples of current and former national bioethics bodies taking such a view are the 1994 National Institutes of Health Human Embryo Research Panel, the National Bioethics Advisory Commission, the U.K. Human Fertilisation and Embryology Authority, and others (see Chapter 4 for elaboration). Unfortunately, the U.S. government has not established such a regulatory system, although many regulations are relevant to these activities, and seems unlikely to do so in the near future, especially in the absence of a substantial federal presence in this field because of the current limitations on the use of federal funding.

However, nonfederally funded hES cell research is going forward in the absence of federal regulation specific to such research, and it is incumbent on the scientific community to exercise the same sort of self-discipline as it has exercised in the past with regard to novel areas of research, such as recombinant DNA in the 1970s. In the absence of a federal regulatory regime designed specifically to provide comprehensive coverage of hES cell research, the committee proposes an oversight system with both local and national components that meets the important goals identified by the other advisory bodies, including the President's Council on Bioethics in its report on NT (President's Council on Bioethics, 2002):

- To support the current consensus against attempts to create children through NT;
- To create a forum for further deliberation on these questions;
- To ensure that legitimate research includes efforts to gather information from animal models and other avenues before utilizing hES cells; and
- To show respect for the deep moral concerns of those who have ethical objections to the research.

RECOMMENDATIONS

Institutional Oversight of hES Cell Research

The ethical and legal concerns involved in hES cell research make increased local oversight by research institutions appropriate. Because of the complexity and novelty of many of the issues involved in hES cell research, the committee believes that all research institutions engaged in hES cell research should create and maintain Embryonic Stem Cell Research Oversight (ESCRO) committees to

1. Provide oversight for all issues related to derivation and use of hES cell lines.
2. Review and approve the scientific merit of research protocols.
3. Review compliance of all in-house hES cell research with all relevant regulations (see Chapter 4) and the guidelines presented in this report (see Chapter 6).
4. Maintain registries of hES cell research conducted at the institution and hES cell lines derived or imported by institutional investigators.
5. Facilitate education of investigators involved in hES cell research.

An ESCRO committee will assist investigators in assessing which regulations might apply to proposed research activities (see Chapter 4 for a fuller discussion). It could serve as a clearinghouse for hES cell research proposals and could assist investigators in identifying the types and levels of review required for a given protocol. For example, the creation of a human/nonhuman chimera may involve review by both an IRB and an Institutional Animal Care and Use Committee (IACUC). In some instances, Institutional Biosafety Committees (IBCs), radiation safety committees, and other groups may also have roles to play in research review (see Chapter 4 for further discussion of the roles of these committees). If hES cell research involves potential clinical applications (such as development of products to be tested in humans), FDA regulations will apply. However, care should be taken that the ESCRO committee does not duplicate or interfere with the proper functions of an IRB or other existing institutional committees. The functions of IRBs and ESCRO committees are distinct and should not be confused.

One particularly important aspect of regulatory compliance for some hES cell research is protection of donors of blastocysts and gametes, which is a matter for IRB review. On the other hand, laboratory research with existing hES cells is generally not covered by federal regulations governing research with human subjects (Department of Health and Human Services [DHHS] regulations at 45 CFR 46, subparts A through D[2]) unless the research involves personally identifiable information about a cell line's progenitors (see Chapter 4). Such research does not need IRB review but should be reviewed by an ESCRO committee. In general, research institutions are likely already to have rules in place for research involving other biological tissues, and, as with any other form of biological or biomedical research, hES cell research would be covered by these rules. But in the case of hES cell research, it will be critically important for investigators and institutions to know the provenance of hES cell lines, particularly if the cell lines are imported to the institution from another site. This would include obtaining an assurance that the process by which the cells were procured was approved by an IRB to ensure that donors provided voluntary informed consent and that risks were minimized (see Chapters 4 and 5). The IRB could be situated at the institution where the cells originated or at the institution where the stem cell research is to be conducted, or it could be independent (non-local). As described in Chapter 5, only one IRB need approve the procurement process, but the institution where the research is to be conducted should obtain evidence of such review. In all cases, the ESCRO committee should

---

[2]DHHS has codified its human subjects protections regulations at 45 CFR 46, subparts A through D. Other agencies have signed onto subpart A, which is referred to as the Common Rule. In this report, DHHS regulations are cited because they are more inclusive than the Common Rule alone, providing protections also to pregnant women, viable fetuses, children, and prisoners. FDA also has codified subpart A of the regulations at 21 CFR 50 and 56 but with slightly different interpretations. In some cases, FDA regulations *and* HHS regulations might apply to research.

ensure that the procurement process has been appropriate by requiring documentation that it was approved by an IRB and adhered to basic principles of ethically responsible procurement. (See Chapter 5 for commentary on requirements for informed consent, payment, timing of consent, and coding of samples.)

The second role of the ESCRO committee is to review research proposals that involve particularly sensitive kinds of research. It is important to note that the vast majority of *in vitro* experiments using already derived hES cell lines are unlikely to raise serious ethical issues and will require minimal review. However, proposals to generate additional hES cell lines by any means will require more extensive review. Some other experiments will also warrant careful consideration, including research in which the identity of the donors of the blastocysts or gametes from which the hES cells were derived is readily ascertainable by the investigator and experiments involving implantation of hES cells or human brain cells into nonhuman animals. Because of the sensitive nature of some aspects of hES cell research, it is critical that the scientific community propose and implement limits on what is to be allowed and provide clear guidance on which research activities require greater scrutiny. Thus, a primary activity of the ESCRO committee will be to ensure that inappropriate research is not conducted and that controversial research is well justified and subject to appropriate additional oversight. Oversight will in many instances conform to a higher standard than is currently required by laws or regulations.

Among those studies that should not be conducted at this time are any that involve *in vitro* culture of any intact human embryo, regardless of derivation method, for longer than 14 days or until formation of the primitive streak begins, whichever occurs first. This is a widely recognized international standard that avoids research on embryos after the formation of the precursors of the brain and central nervous system. Research in which hES cells are introduced into nonhuman primate blastocysts, or in which animal or human ES cells are introduced into human blastocysts, should also not be conducted at this time. These kinds of studies could produce creatures in which the lines between human and nonhuman primates are blurred, a development that could threaten to undermine human dignity. Finally, although it is unlikely, hES cells introduced into nonhuman hosts might be able to generate gametes, so any such human/nonhuman chimeras should not be allowed to breed (see Chapter 2 for further discussion). In all those cases, future scientific advances might render the concerns moot or might raise new concerns, so the category of currently nonpermissible experiments will need review in the future (see later discussion of a national review panel).

The ESCRO committee must have suitable scientific, medical, and ethical expertise to conduct its own review and should have the resources needed to coordinate the management of the various other reviews that may be required for a particular protocol. Besides scientists and ethicists, its membership should also include at least one person from the community. A pre-existing committee could serve the functions of the ESCRO committee provided that it has the recommended expertise and representation to perform the various roles described in this report.

For example, an institution might elect to constitute an ESCRO committee from among some members of an IRB. But the ESCRO committee should not be a subcommittee of the IRB, as its responsibilities extend beyond human subject protections. Furthermore, much hES cell research does not require IRB review.

Because stem cell research is subject to a greater degree of public interest and scrutiny than most other laboratory and clinical research, the committee believes that each institution should maintain through its ESCRO committee a registry of hES cell lines in use and of investigators working with them and descriptive information on the types of hES cell research in which they are engaged. The purposes of such a registry include facilitating distribution of educational information in light of evolving ethical, legal, or regulatory issues and enabling an institution to respond to public inquiry about the extent of its involvement in hES cell research. The ESCRO committee should also play a central role in educating investigators—including research staff, fellows, and students—on ethical, legal, and policy issues in stem cell research. That might include developing and maintaining a web-based primer, such as those commonly used at research institutions that support human subjects research.

The foregoing concerns give rise to the following recommendations.

Recommendation 1:

To provide local oversight of all issues related to derivation and research use of hES cell lines and to facilitate education of investigators involved in hES cell research, all institutions conducting hES cell research should establish an Embryonic Stem Cell Research Oversight (ESCRO) committee. The committee should include representatives of the public and persons with expertise in developmental biology, stem cell research, molecular biology, assisted reproduction, and ethical and legal issues in hES cell research. The ESCRO committee would not substitute for an Institutional Review Board but rather would provide an additional level of review and scrutiny warranted by the complex issues raised by hES cell research. The committee would also serve to review basic hES cell research using preexisting anonymous cell lines that does not require consideration by an Institutional Review Board.

Recommendation 2:

Through its Embryonic Stem Cell Research Oversight (ESCRO) committee, each research institution should ensure that the provenance of hES cells is documented. Documentation should include evidence that the procurement process was approved by an Institutional Review Board to ensure adherence to the basic ethical and legal principles of informed consent and protection of confidentiality.

Recommendation 3:
Embryonic Stem Cell Research Oversight (ESCRO) committees or their equivalents should divide research proposals into three categories in setting limits on research and determining the requisite level of oversight:

(a) Research that is permissible after notification of the research institution's ESCRO committee and completion of the reviews mandated by current requirements. Purely *in vitro* hES cell research with pre-existing coded or anonymous hES cell lines in general is permissible provided that notice of the research, documentation of the provenance of the cell lines, and evidence of compliance with any required Institutional Review Board, Institutional Animal Care and Use Committee, Institutional Biosafety Committee, or other mandated reviews is provided to the ESCRO committee or other body designated by the investigator's institution.

(b) Research that is permissible only after additional review and approval by an ESCRO committee or other equivalent body designated by the investigator's institution.
> (i) The ESCRO committee should evaluate all requests for permission to attempt derivation of new hES cell lines from donated blastocysts, from *in vitro* fertilized oocytes, or by nuclear transfer. The scientific rationale for the need to generate new hES cell lines, by whatever means, must be clearly presented, and the basis for the numbers of blastocysts and oocytes needed should be justified. Such requests should be accompanied by evidence of Institutional Review Board approval of the procurement process.
> (ii) All research involving the introduction of hES cells into nonhuman animals at any stage of embryonic, fetal, or postnatal development should be reviewed by the ESCRO committee. Particular attention should be paid to the probable pattern and effects of differentiation and integration of the human cells into the nonhuman animal tissues.
> (iii) Research in which personally identifiable information about the donors of the blastocysts, gametes, or somatic cells from which the hES cells were derived is readily ascertainable by the investigator also requires ESCRO committee review and approval.

(c) Research that should not be permitted at this time:
> (i) Research involving *in vitro* culture of any intact human embryo, regardless of derivation method, for longer than 14 days or until formation of the primitive streak begins, whichever occurs first.
> (ii) Research in which hES cells are introduced into nonhuman primate blastocysts or in which any ES cells are introduced into human blastocysts.

In addition:
     (iii) No animal into which hES cells have been introduced at any stage of development should be allowed to breed.

Recommendation 4:
Through its Embryonic Stem Cell Research Oversight (ESCRO) committee, each research institution should establish and maintain a registry of investigators conducting hES cell research and record descriptive information about the types of research being performed and the hES cells in use.

Investigators who collaborate across national boundaries should respect the ethical standards and procedural protections applicable in all the relevant jurisdictions.

Recommendation 5:
If a U.S.-based investigator collaborates with an investigator in another country, the Embryonic Stem Cell Research Oversight (ESCRO) committee may determine that the procedures prescribed by the foreign institution afford protections equivalent with these guidelines and may approve the substitution of some or all of the foreign procedures for its own.

The committee hesitates to recommend another bureaucratic entity to oversee the biomedical research system, but in this case it believes the burden to be justified because of the special issues involved in hES cell research and the diverse entities that might have a role in the review process in a research institution. A coordination function is crucial. In some cases, smaller institutions may wish to avail themselves of the services of larger facilities that have ESCRO committees.

The creation of an ESCRO committee to perform functions unique to hES cell oversight does not relieve institutions or scientific investigators, regardless of their field, of the ultimate responsibility to ensure that they conduct themselves in accordance with professional standards and integrity. In particular, people whose research involves hES cells should work closely with oversight bodies, demonstrate respect for the autonomy and privacy of those who donate gametes and embryos, and be sensitive to public concerns about research involving human embryos.

Need for a National Perspective

As individual states and private entities move into the field of hES cell research, it is important to initiate a national effort to provide a formal context in which the complex moral and oversight questions associated with this work can be addressed. The state of the science of hES cell research and the clinical practice and public policy surrounding these topics are in a state of flux and are likely to be so for several years. Therefore, the committee believes that some entity needs to be established to review the policies and guidelines covering appropriate practices in this field but not to review and approve specific research protocols, an activity that will best occur at the local institutional level. Such national bodies have been established in most other countries where hES cell research has been debated and approved—such as Australia, Canada, Israel, Singapore, and the United Kingdom (see Chapter 4)—usually under government auspices. Some of those bodies also have responsibility for reviewing individual research proposals, and such centralized review entities may serve well in smaller jurisdictions where public funds are being used in the research. However, in line with the longstanding practice in the United States of using local review boards for human subjects research, animal research, and biohazards, the committee believes that local review of individual research proposals by ESCRO committees (with involvement of IRBs, IACUCs, IBCs, and other panels as described above) will be the best mechanism of oversight of hES cell research. Nonetheless, there will be a need for continuing consideration of new issues that arise from scientific advances, clinical applications, or public policy concerns that will need to be discussed in a central forum. Such a forum should from time to time review the adequacy of the guidelines proposed in this report (Chapter 6) in light of changes in science and the emergence of new issues of public interest. New policies and standards may be appropriate for issues that cannot currently be foreseen.

The organization that sponsors the public forum should be one that is respected in the lay and scientific communities, is politically independent without conflicts of interest, and is able to call on suitable expertise to support the effort. Its membership should include nationally and internationally recognized authorities in the scientific, medical, ethical, and legal issues associated with hES cell research, and representatives of the public. The proposed national body must pay careful attention to evidence and argumentation in its deliberations, as well as taking into account the diverse views of the public on these sensitive and evolving issues.

To help ensure that these guidelines are taken seriously, the various stakeholders in hES cell research—sponsors, funding sources, research institutions, relevant oversight committees, professional societies, and scientific journals, as well as investigators—should develop policies and practices that are consistent with these guidelines and adhere to the recommendations of the national panel. Funding agencies, professional societies, journals, and institutional review panels can provide valuable community pressure and sanctions to ensure compliance. For example, ESCRO committees and IRBs should require evidence of compliance when protocols are reviewed for renewal, funding agencies should assess compliance when reviewing applications for support, and journals should require that evidence of compliance accompanies publication of results.

Recommendation 6:
A national body should be established to assess periodically the adequacy of the guidelines proposed in this document and to provide a forum for a continuing discussion of issues involved in hES cell research.

The Just Distribution of the Benefits of hES Cell Research

Billions of dollars will be committed to hES cell research from public and private sources in the coming years. It is not yet clear exactly what specific therapeutic benefits will emerge from this investment, but there is reason for concern that they will not be equitably distributed in our current health-care system. Skeptics may argue that the social investment in science that still requires much research before any health benefits will be realized is not merited when so many basic, often technology-intensive, health services are not adequately provided.

The therapeutic possibilities inherent in hES cells can mean vastly improved lives for millions of disease sufferers, and the successful practice of regenerative medicine could yield substantial reductions in health-care expenditures. It is critical that hES cell research, especially as it approaches clinical application, serve the needs of all populations. There must be a concerted effort to ensure diversity not just in the genetic makeup of cell lines but in the approaches to clinical care. Our current health-care system is not well designed for the just distribution of the benefits of research. Besides the excellent scientific work that will surely be accomplished, institutions involved in hES cell research should concern themselves with ensuring genetic diversity in the development of cell lines and in devising health-care systems that can make the long-term benefits of this work widely available.

Recommendation 7:
The hES cell research community should ensure that there is sufficient genetic diversity among cell lines to allow for potential translation into health-care services for all groups in our society.

CONCLUSION

The proposed local ESCRO committees and national forum should help to ensure that conventional and well founded research practices and protections apply to hES cell research. Among those practices is the use of *in vitro* and animal models before interventions that involve human subjects. Protections include minimizing the use of human gametes or embryos and ensuring that recruitment, disclosure, informed consent, and risk assessment procedures are in accord with the highest ethical standards. The consensus on prohibition of NT for reproductive purposes can also be reinforced with a rigorous system of oversight of hES cell research. With this system in place, the scientific community will signal its respect for the views of those who have ethical reservations about the research and provide an opportunity for those views to be expressed. As some have observed, when many people find a practice morally troubling—particularly one that is novel—that is an indication that further consideration is required. An initial reaction of moral alarm need not be decisive. Many practices that are now regarded as morally noncontroversial, such as blood transfusions, organ transplants and *in vitro* fertilization, were once seen by many as shocking and unacceptable; others that are now regarded as unacceptable, such as blood-letting, were conventional. Moral perceptions are sharpened with experience, through the growth of knowledge, and the consideration of various viewpoints. Even if the underlying principles do not change, the interpretation and application of the principles often do.

The next chapter addresses the specific regulatory issues that might apply to hES cell research.

4

Current Regulation of
Human Embryonic Stem Cell Research

It would be a mistake to assume that the restrictions on federal funding for human embryonic stem (hES) cell research result in an absence of oversight of such work. At present, many federal regulations already govern various aspects of hES cell research, including

- Human subjects protection for donors of somatic cells and oocytes and for some donors of embryos.
- Medical privacy protections.
- Laboratory standards for investigators whose work will result in products that require Food and Drug Administration (FDA) approval.
- Safety reviews of laboratory work that involves genetic alteration of hES cell lines.
- Animal care committee reviews of hES cell research that uses nonhuman animals.
- Various rules governing the importation of biological materials or the transfer of medical data from other countries.

However, there is a perception that the field is unregulated. In fact, the field is subject to a patchwork of regulations, many not designed with this research specifically in mind, and the patchwork has some gaps in its coverage.

This chapter reviews current state and federal regulation of hES cell research in the United States, noting where gaps in regulatory coverage are addressed by the guidelines proposed later in this report (Chapter 6). It also offers some examples of how the proposed guidelines would operate in conjunction with current regulations and presents comparisons with regulations in other nations that have substantial hES cell research programs. Recommendations about the application of existing regulatory conventions to hES cell research are offered.

Finally, although the committee recognizes that successful resolution of intellectual property issues will be critically important in this evolving area of research, it was beyond its charge and beyond its capabilities to address adequately all of the legal issues that will arise. In the context of privately funded research it is particularly difficult to explore mechanisms by which discoveries made using hES cells can be made widely accessible for the benefit of human health. However, the committee believes that best practices can be developed and followed. Several policy statements developed regarding patenting and licensing issues more generally applied in biomedical science can serve as aspirational goals for the hES cell research community. In particular, in 2004 NIH issued *Best Practices for the Licensing of Genomic Inventions.*[1] This document aims to maximize the public benefit whenever Public Health Service-owned or -funded technologies are transferred to the commercial sector. In this document NIH recommends that "whenever possible, non-exclusive licensing should be pursued as a best practice. A non-exclusive licensing approach favors and facilitates making broad enabling technologies and research uses of inventions widely available and accessible to the scientific community." In addition, the National Academies is developing recommendations for NIH on intellectual property rights in genomic- and protein-related innovation (forthcoming, 2005). The reader is encouraged to review these documents, which aim to facilitate responsible patenting and licensing practices by the scientific community.

REGULATION OF PROCUREMENT OF GAMETES, SOMATIC CELLS, AND BLASTOCYSTS

Whether it involves receiving donated blastocysts that would otherwise be discarded after infertility treatment or procuring gametes and somatic cells to make blastocysts specifically for research purposes, the procurement process often requires oversight by an Institutional Review Board (IRB), whose membership and functions are described in Department of Health and Human Service (DHHS) regulations at 45 CFR 46.107-115 and in FDA regulations at 21 CFR 56.107-115.[2] IRB

---

[1]http://a257.g.akamaitech.net/7/257/2422/06jun20041800/edocket.access.gpo.gov/2004/pdf/04-25671.pdf.

[2]DHHS has codified its human subjects protection regulations at 45 CFR 46, Subparts A through D. Other federal research agencies have signed onto Subpart A, which is referred to as the Common Rule. In this report, the DHHS regulations are cited in discussing the protection of human subjects of research because they are more inclusive than the Common Rule alone. The DHHS regulations extend additional protections to vulnerable populations, such as pregnant women, viable fetuses, prisoners, and children. FDA also has codified Subpart A of the regulations at 21 CFR 50 and 56, although with slightly different interpretations. In some cases, FDA regulations and HHS regulations might apply to research.

review is the primary means of implementing the research protections found in the federal regulations, which generally require that human research be undertaken with the informed and voluntary consent of the subjects, that the risks to subjects be minimized, and that the research be approved and monitored by an IRB. The federal regulations generally are triggered when research is funded by the federal government, when privately funded research is aimed at developing data for a product to be approved by FDA, or when privately funded research takes place at institutions that have agreed to adopt the protections more broadly than required by law. In addition, some states, such as California and New Jersey, have adopted legislation requiring IRB review and many of the substantive protections of the federal regulations with regard to hES cell research conducted in those states.[3]

Research involving hES cells will require access to human oocytes and blastocysts, which in turn will necessitate some interaction between donors of oocytes and blastocysts and the people or institutions seeking to procure these materials for use in hES cell research. The federal regulations governing human subjects research define human subjects research as involving either

(1) obtaining data from a living individual through intervention or interaction with the individual; or
(2) obtaining private (i.e., individually identifiable) information about a living individual (45 CFR 46.102(f)).

The DHHS Office for Human Research Protections (OHRP) has made it clear that hES cell research "that involves neither interactions nor interventions with living individuals or obtaining identifiable private information is not considered human subjects research [and therefore] IRB review is not required for such research."[4] According to OHRP, merely asking couples whether they wish to donate their surplus blastocysts for research does not render them "human subjects of research" if no data on them are being gathered and there is no substantive interaction with them other than gaining their consent.[5]

On the other hand, where physical interaction is needed to obtain biological materials, such as in the case of donors whose sperm, oocytes, or somatic cells are used to make blastocysts for research, the interaction brings them under the purview of the human subjects protections system and IRB review is required, even though the donors are not themselves the subjects of scientific study. Thus, their fully informed and voluntary consent is required before such research use.

---

[3]See http://www.ncsl.org/programs/health/genetics/rt-shcl.htm.
[4]*Guidance for Investigators and Institutional Review Boards Regarding Human Embryonic Stem Cells, Germ Cells and Stem Cell-Derived Test Articles,* OHRP/DHHS, Mar. 19, 2002, at 3.
[5]OHRP staff briefing to the committee, January 8, 2005, interpreting 45 CFR 46.102(f).

Whether it is blastocyst donation or the donation of gametes and somatic cells, even where the federal regulations require informed consent, IRBs are permitted to waive the requirement if certain conditions are met (45 CFR 46. 116(8)(d)), that is, if the research is of minimal risk, waiver of consent would not adversely affect rights and welfare of subjects, and obtaining consent is impracticable. In the case of gamete or somatic cell donation, in which the donors must be present at the time of donation, not all those conditions apply, and waiver of consent cannot be granted. In the case of blastocyst donation, the committee finds that informed consent should be required in all cases (see Chapter 5): a waiver should not be granted even when the specified conditions can be met.

Although OHRP requires IRB review of the procurement process for blastocyst donors only under certain conditions, this committee finds that the best way to ensure that protections are in place for all potential donors is to require IRB review at all times for the process by which somatic cells, gametes, and blastocysts are obtained to ensure that risks are minimized and voluntary and informed consent is provided. (Consent issues are addressed in greater detail in Chapter 5.) In contrast, as noted below in the discussion of privacy protections, when research is to be conducted on hES cell lines that have already been derived through a procurement process approved by an IRB, the committee does not find that there is need for additional IRB review of work with coded or anonymous cell lines.

Recommendation 8:
Regardless of the source of funding and the applicability of federal regulations, an Institutional Review Board or its equivalent should review the procurement of gametes, blastocysts, or somatic cells for the purpose of generating new hES cell lines, including the procurement of blastocysts in excess of clinical need from *in vitro* fertilization clinics, blastocysts made through *in vitro* fertilization specifically for research purposes, and oocytes, sperm, and somatic cells donated for development of hES cell lines derived through nuclear transfer.

Recommendation 9:
Institutional Review Boards may not waive the requirement for obtaining informed consent from any person whose somatic cells, gametes, or blastocysts are used in hES research.

Requiring informed consent before donation of gametes, somatic cells, or blastocysts and requiring oversight by such a body as an IRB would bring U.S. practices into conformity with the practices in Australia, Canada, Israel, Singapore, the United Kingdom, and other major centers of hES cell research. That, in turn, will not only ensure the ethical conduct of procurement practices in the United States but also facilitate collaboration with investigators subject to regulations in the other countries.

THE PRIVACY RULE AND HUMAN SUBJECTS PROTECTIONS FOR RESEARCH WITH BIOLOGICAL MATERIALS: IMPLICATIONS FOR hES CELL RESEARCH

In many cases, medical information about donors will be collected at the time of gamete or blastocyst donation. The primary purpose of collecting such information is to permit a coded link to be maintained between the resulting hES cell lines and information about the genetic or infectious disease status of the donors. The information could facilitate some types of research (such as genetics research) or might be needed to enhance suitability screening for downstream tissue transplantation uses (see later discussion of FDA donor suitability rules).

How such donor information is collected and managed can affect whether the human subjects protections described above apply and whether federal privacy protections apply. Thus, a key determinant is whether the resulting cell lines will be managed in a way that makes the donors' identities readily ascertainable to investigators. If so, both sets of protections apply.

When investigators wish to work with existing lines rather than obtain materials to derive new lines, those lines may be accompanied by medical or other information about the donors. Work with hES cell lines whose identifiers render identity of the original donors readily ascertainable to the investigators would be a form of human subjects research that requires IRB review because the work might well reveal information about the donors. But properly obscuring donor identities can exempt work with cell lines from the requirement of IRB review. In that situation, OHRP has declared that *in vitro* research or research in animals that involves the use of an hES cell line that "retains a link to identifying [donor] information" (such as the use of a code) will not be considered human subjects research subject to the federal regulations if

(1) the investigator and research institution do not have access to identifiable private information related to the cell line; and

(2) a written agreement is obtained from the holder of the identifiable private information related to the cell line providing that such information will not be released to the investigator under any circumstances.[6]

OHRP has stated that, when those two conditions are satisfied, the research is not considered to involve human subjects, because the donors' identities cannot be readily ascertained by the investigator or associated with the cell line. By necessary implication, the OHRP *Guidance* dictates that any hES cell researcher who has access to personally identifiable information regarding the donors, including medi-

---

[6]See also *Guidance on Research Involving Coded Private Information or Biological Specimens*, OHRP/DHHS, Aug. 10, 2004.

cal information, will fall within the regulatory purview, and IRB review will be required. Thus, when medical information required for FDA donor suitability rules is collected (see below), human subjects protections are triggered unless the information is carefully coded and managed.

In addition to human subjects protections, if donor health information is attached to hES cell lines, federal privacy protections under the Health Insurance Portability and Accountability Act of 1996 (HIPAA; PL 104-191) might apply. The Privacy Rule of HIPAA might be applicable to hES cell research if the investigator obtains personal health information (PHI) on donors and the investigator is a "covered entity" (most likely a provider that transmits information in electronic format, such as a physician or hospital).[7] The Privacy Rule would permit PHI obtained by the researcher to be "deidentified," for example, statistical data would be aggregated or stripped of individual identifiers (45 CFR 164.514(b)) so that it could be used or disclosed without restriction.

If an hES cell investigator is employed by a covered entity and does not wish to "deidentify" PHI related to donors of somatic cells, gametes, or blastocysts (presumably because the identifying information may be expected to contribute relevant scientific information or assist in FDA review), HIPAA requires either of these

- A valid "authorization" from the donor before the PHI is used or disclosed (45 CFR 164.508).
- Appropriate documentation that an IRB or a privacy board has granted a waiver or alteration of the authorization requirement that satisfies 45 CFR 164.512(i).[8]

The criteria for approving an authorization waiver or alteration must be consistent with the criteria for IRB waiver of the informed consent:

(1) PHI is protected by a plan to guard against unauthorized disclosure, so there is no more than "minimal risk" to privacy;

2) The research could not practicably be conducted without the requested waiver or alteration; and

3) The research could not practicably be conducted without access to and use of the PHI (45 CFR164.512(i)(2)(ii)(A)-(C)).

---

[7]See 65 Fed. Reg. 82,799 (Dec. 28, 2000) (defining *covered entities*).

[8]An example of a situation in which a waiver of authorization requirements may be deemed appropriate by an IRB is a study that involves the use of PHI on numerous people whose contact information is unknown. The research would be impracticable to conduct if authorization were required, and an IRB could waive all the authorization requirements if the waiver criteria were satisfied. If the IRB approves such a waiver, the receipt of the requisite documentation of the approval permits a covered entity to use or disclose PHI in connection with a particular research project without authorization.

In sum, FDA's donor suitability rules (discussed below) may require collection of medical record information on donors of somatic cells, gametes, or blastocysts whose biological materials were used to derive new hES cell lines. In such cases, both federal human subjects protections and the Privacy Rule might apply to the research uses of the information, depending on how it is collected and transmitted in conjunction with the cell lines. Thus, if hES cell research involves the transmission of PHI on the donors, which will increasingly be the case as cell lines approach clinical application, it will be important for investigators, institutions, and IRBs to be aware of any Privacy Rule requirements that apply and to seek authorization from donors, as appropriate, for the transmission of health information.

Recommendation 10:

Investigators, institutions, Institutional Review Boards, and privacy boards should ensure that authorizations are received from donors, as appropriate and required by federal human subjects protections and the Health Insurance Portability and Accountability Act, for the confidential transmission of personal health information to repositories or to investigators who are using hES cell lines derived from donated materials.

REGULATION OF *IN VITRO* AND ANIMAL STUDIES THAT USE hES CELL LINES

In general, state law does not affect the practice of *in vitro* or animal studies with hES cells. There are, however, sources of federal regulation for this research.

Once the cell lines are established, as noted above, federal regulations governing human research and HIPAA regulations apply only if information being used or developed might personally identify the original donors and progenitors. Thus, *in vitro* or animal studies that use hES cell lines do not require IRB review if the tracking codes that link the donors to the cell lines are properly managed. However, a host of other federal regulations apply to even purely laboratory, preclinical research with hES cell lines.

Recombinant DNA Research

Some of the research being done on hES cell lines will require some degree of genetic manipulation (see Chapter 2 for a description of these experiments). Research institutions are responsible for ensuring that all recombinant DNA research conducted at or sponsored by them is conducted in compliance with the National Institutes of Health *Guidelines for Research Involving Recombinant DNA Molecules*.[9] Institutional authority and responsibility place accountability for the safe

---

[9]Available at http://www4.od.nih.gov/oba/rac/guidelines/guidelines.html.

conduct of such research at the local level, and oversight is managed through an Institutional Biosafety Committee (IBC), a review body registered with NIH and appointed by an institution to review and approve potentially biohazardous lines of research.[10]

The need for IBCs grew out of the Asilomar Conference, when scientists agreed to self-regulate recombinant DNA research to avoid any potential threats to human health or the environment. Much of that research was initially reviewed case-by-case, not only by IBCs but also by a federal-level committee, the Recombinant DNA Advisory Committee (RAC). Over time RAC's role has evolved, first toward a focus on human gene transfer therapy study approvals and more recently toward human gene transfer therapy policy development, with authority to approve gene transfer therapy studies lodged solely in FDA's jurisdiction. To the extent possible, review of individual recombinant DNA research proposals has been delegated to local IBCs, and they remain as the guardians of public safety with regard to all recombinant DNA research and other potentially biohazardous research. They focus their review on safety, not on compliance with human subjects protections or other aspects of state and federal law governing the ethical conduct of scientific research. Many experiments are reviewed and approved by IBCs without any input from RAC.

At present, RAC is an advisory committee whose goal is to consider the current state of knowledge and technology regarding recombinant DNA. This includes review but not approval of human gene transfer trials, and assessment of the ability of DNA recombinants to survive in nature and the potential for transfer of genetic material to other organisms. A major role for RAC is to examine clinical trials that involve the transfer of recombinant DNA to humans. Currently, all human gene transfer trials in which NIH funding is involved (either directly or indirectly) are registered with the RAC. Protocols that contain unique and/or novel issues are discussed in a public forum. In addition, RAC advises the NIH director and his/her staff in a number of activities, including the preparation of materials required in legal actions, international coordination of biotechnology regulations, and the review of regulations proposed by other federal agencies.

In contrast to RAC's role, FDA's role is to determine whether a sponsor may begin studying a gene transfer product and, ultimately, whether it is safe and effective for human use. FDA regulates the products evaluated in human gene transfer clinical trials that are intended for eventual sale in the United States and is responsible for reviewing serious adverse events that occur in a gene transfer study.

Animal Care and Use

Increasingly, hES cell research might also involve the manipulation of hES cells in a nonhuman animal, such as a mouse. Laboratory work with nonhuman animals

---

[10]See http://www4.od.nih.gov/oba/IBC/IBCrole.htm.

is governed by its own set of federal laws and regulations, and any hES cell research that involves insertion of hES cells or their derivatives into animals is already subject to animal welfare protections. The Animal Welfare Act constitutes congressional policy to ensure the most humane use of animals in research. Some animals that might be used by hES cell investigators are not covered by the act, but most are covered.[11] In addition, the Public Health Service (PHS) Policy on Humane Care and Use of Laboratory Animals requires that each institution receiving PHS support for an activity involving any live vertebrate animals establish an appropriate institutional animal care and use program, including an Institutional Animal Care and Use Committee (IACUC) with specific responsibilities as described in the PHS policy.[12]

Laboratory Practice

In addition to special regulations governing recombinant DNA research and research that uses animals, the federal government has regulations pertaining to the management of laboratories where products that might ultimately be introduced into humans (as in a clinical trial) are being developed. FDA's Good Laboratory Practice (GLP) regulations establish standards for nonclinical laboratory studies. These do not include basic exploratory studies performed to determine whether a test article has any potential utility or to determine its physical or chemical characteristics but they do encompass *in vivo* or *in vitro* experiments in which test articles are studied to determine their safety—an activity that would be characteristic of the preclinical phase of hES cell research. Failure to conform to GLP regulations, although not itself a violation of law, would render any hES cells less useful in the future if they were considered for clinical trials of tissue transplantation or other cell-based therapies.[13]

Recommendation 11:
Investigators and institutions involved in hES cell research should conduct the research in accordance with all applicable laws and guidelines pertaining to recombinant DNA research and animal care. Institutions should consider adopting Good Laboratory Practice standards for some or all of their basic hES cell research.

REGULATION OF CLINICAL RESEARCH WITH CELL LINES AND DIFFERENTIATED TISSUE

Clinical research aimed at obtaining FDA approval or new labeling of drugs, devices, or biologics is subject to regulation by FDA. It must be conducted in

---

[11]Animal Welfare Act (as amended), 7 USC §§ 2131-56.

[12]http://grants.nih.gov/grants/olaw/references/phspol.htm.

[13]http://www.fda.gov/ora/compliance_ref/bimo/7348_808/part_I.html.

compliance with FDA's regulations governing investigational new drugs (INDs) or investigational device exemptions (IDEs), regardless of source of funding. Thus, all human studies conducted under INDs and IDEs are subject to FDA's own regulations concerning IRB review and informed consent (21 CFR 50 and 56), which are roughly parallel to the DHHS regulations at 45 CFR 46.

Transplantation of hES cells or tissues developed from hES cell lines is a form of "cell-based therapy" and is generally regulated by FDA as a biologic, drug, or device. The regulations entail a variety of premarket notifications and approvals based on safety and efficacy data; the precise requirements depend on the primary mode of action (drug or device), in accordance with the Food, Drug and Cosmetic Act and its amendments (21 USC Section 301 *et seq*). Biologics are subject to additional precautions based on the Public Health Service Act, aimed primarily at control of transmission of infectious disease (42 USC, Chapter 6A, Part F).

Because hES cell research is likely to lead to clinical applications that involve the transfer of cells or tissue into humans they will also be subject to FDA's comprehensive tissue transplantation regulations.[14] Of course, many investigators will be engaged in basic research with no intent to pursue an immediate clinical application, and much of what follows does not necessarily apply to such investigators. But failure to follow FDA's tissue transplantation regulations may result in FDA's refusal to use materials from the laboratories in question in later clinical trials. If so, investigators might have to derive new cell lines in accordance with the regulations if their materials are to be acceptable for development into transplantable tissue.

FDA's new, more comprehensive approach to regulating tissue transplantation was announced in February 1997.[15] Although only partially implemented as of 2005, FDA already requires registration by all establishments that recover, process, store, label, package, or distribute "human cells, tissues, and cellular and tissue-based products" (HCT/Ps) or that screen or test donors of them. The registration requirement is applicable to establishments involved in the derivation and management of hES cell lines and resulting tissues that will be used for transplantation into humans.

In addition, as of May 2005, FDA's "current good tissue practices" (CGTP) will include rules governing the process for procuring human blastocysts, oocytes, sperm, and somatic cells for use in research leading to clinical applications. The rules will include donor screening to prevent the spread of communicable diseases and a tracking system that will permit tracking from each human cell line or tissue back to the original donor. For work with existing cell lines, CGTP rules already govern the methods and facilities used for the manufacture of HCT/Ps to prevent the introduction or transmission of communicable diseases by these cells, tissues, and products. As with the registration requirements, the rules apply to HCT/Ps that are destined for transplantation into humans.

---

[14]http://www.fda.gov/cber/tissue/tissue.htm.
[15]http://www.fda.gov/cber/tissue/tissue.htm.

Once a donation has been made, the resulting tissue must be coded in a fashion that permits tracking back to the original donor if that is needed, and a summary of relevant information about the donor must accompany the cell line or tissue whenever it is passed to a new facility.[16]

Because those rules require some kind of tracking system that will maintain a connection between the donor and the endproduct, such as transplantable tissue, the FDA tissue rules have an effect on the operation of human subjects protections, as well as the HIPAA Privacy Rule. The net effects are that

- Work on completely anonymous hES cell lines will not be human subjects research, but this tissue may well be disfavored by FDA if investigators wish to use it for clinical trials. FDA will prefer that trials use tissue for which there is a traceable history back to the donors and their medical histories.
- Work on hES cell lines with identifiers linking them to the donors will be subject to federal regulations governing human subjects research and, in the case of covered entities, HIPAA privacy protections unless the identifiers are coded and managed in a fashion that renders the donors effectively unidentifiable to the investigators.

Finally, work with hES cell lines that were grown on mouse feeder cells may face a special obstacle if an investigator wishes to use them to develop transplantable tissue for human clinical trials. FDA's regulations define xenotransplantation to include any procedure that involves the transplantation of human body fluids, cells, tissues or organs that have had *ex vivo* contact with live nonhuman animal cells, tissues, or organs. Tissue transplantation from cell lines grown on nonhuman feeder cells would be considered xenotransplantation and would require additional FDA review.[17]

For hES cell investigators who plan to obtain cell lines from outside the United States, it is worth noting that FDA's new tissue regulations also govern the importation of cell lines and derived tissues for use in clinical transplantation, and importation must be approved by FDA, whose regulations pursuant to Section 361 of the Public Health Service Act are designed to prevent the transmission of communicable diseases.

Also of relevance to researchers working with cell lines from other countries, there are medical privacy requirements in other countries that must be considered whenever transnational collaborations are contemplated.[18] For collaborations with

---

[16]See § 1271.55 of the new regulations, as presented in "Eligibility Determination for Donors of Human Cells, Tissues, and Cellular and Tissue-Based Products", *Federal Register* Vol. 69, No. 101, amending 21 CFR Parts 210, 211, 820, and 1271, 69 FR 29786 (May 25, 2004).

[17]http://www.fda.gov/cber/xap/xap.htm.

[18]"New International Guidelines on the Transfer of Personal Health Data," William R. M. Long and Julia Barnes, *Medical Research & Policy News*, Volume 4 Number 4, February 16, 2005 Page 157, ISSN 1539-4530.

members of the European Union, Iceland, Liechtenstein, and Norway, medical information about donors that accompanies cell lines must comply with the guidelines issued by the International Organisation for Standardisation (ISO).[19] Those rules generally preclude the transfer of medical data about identifiable persons unless consent has been obtained and the country receiving the data has an adequate system for medical data protection.[20] Despite the passage of HIPAA, the United States has not been deemed to have such a system, although individual institutions may devise systems that meet the European requirements.

Many forms of hES cell research, however, can be exempted from the rules, provided that the data are rendered anonymous. Under the ISO guidelines, anonymization means rendering data "nonpersonal," that is, the codes do not directly or indirectly reveal the identity of the donors.[21] Given the varied ways in which anonymous is interpreted under HIPAA, ISO guidelines, and federal human subjects research rules, investigators and institutions need to be attentive to the concerns of all appropriate bodies before working with cell lines that are understood to be anonymized.

Recommendation 12:
hES cell research leading to potential clinical application must be in compliance with all applicable Food and Drug Administration (FDA) regulations. If FDA requires that a link to the donor source be maintained, investigators and institutions must ensure that the confidentiality of the donor is protected, that the donor understands that a link will be maintained, and that, where applicable, federal human subjects protections and Health Insurance Portability and Accountability Act or other privacy protections are followed.

U.S. STATE LAW ON hES CELL RESEARCH

State law rarely addresses the regulation of medical research. It does, however, often address the status of embryos. In this respect, it is relevant to hES cell research.

---

[19]ISO 22857: 2004(E)—"Health informatics—Guidelines on data protection to facilitate trans-border flows of personal health information."

[20]The ISO guidelines are based on four other pieces of transnational legislation: "Recommendations of the Council of the OECD concerning Guidelines on the Protection of Privacy and Trans-border flows of Personal Data" [OECD, Sept. 23, 1980, and "Guidelines for the Security of Information Systems," OECD, 1996.]; the "Council of Europe Recommendation R(97)5 on the Protection of Medical Data" (Council of Europe Publishing, Strasbourg, Feb. 12, 1997); actions of the U.N. General Assembly, Dec. 14, 1990; and the EU Data Protection Directive (Directive 95/46/EC of the European Parliament and of the Council of Oct. 24, 1995, on the protection of individuals with regard to the processing of personal data and on the free movement of such data. OJL 281, Nov. 23, 1995, p. 31). The latter directive was last amended by Regulation (EC) No. 1882/2003 of the European Parliament and of the Council of Sept. 29, 2003, OJL 289, Oct. 31, 2003, p. 1.

[21]Recital 26 of the EU Data Protection Directive provides that the principles of protection shall not apply to data rendered anonymous in such a way that the data subject is no longer identifiable.

Courts have held that dispositional authority over an embryo in general belongs to the progenitors.[22] Moreover, case law suggests that destruction of an embryo does not require the consent of anonymous gamete donors, although in the context of couples who disagreed over the disposition of embryos, the consent of both partners has been required before release of an embryo for reproductive purposes, particularly in the absence of a prior agreement between the partners.[23] In the absence of a joint decision regarding disposition, however, current law will result in leaving the embryo in a frozen state. Fertility clinics have sought to avoid such conflicts by asking couples to agree in advance on the terms on which embryos can be released for reproductive use, kept frozen, discarded, or released for research.

A number of states, such as Louisiana, Maine, Massachusetts, Minnesota, New Hampshire, North Dakota, Pennsylvania, and Rhode Island, have enacted legislation to prohibit or limit research with human embryos,[24] with the definition of embryo occasionally merged with the definition of fetus.[25] In some cases, these state laws restricting embryo research have been challenged successfully in court, on grounds such as unconstitutional vagueness.[26] But most U.S. states have no laws or regulations specifically addressing hES cell research. Of the laws that do exist, many focus exclusively on nuclear transfer (NT) research. For example, as of March 2005, Arkansas, Iowa, Michigan, North Dakota, and South Dakota had laws that clearly forbid the use of NT for research purposes.[27] Missouri forbids the use of state funds for NT research.[28] Other states, such as Rhode Island and Virginia (less clear from the text of the law), have banned NT for reproductive purposes but have not addressed its use for research purposes.[29] In states that do not forbid NT research, it remains legal and subject to the federal regulations described above. New Jersey and California, however, have adopted laws that add extra state regulation to the field of hES cell and NT research, most notably by expanding the jurisdiction of IRBs to review the research and by prohibiting the sale of embryos.[30] In California, however, research funded pursuant to the Proposition 71 initiative will be exempt

[22]See York v. Jones, 717 F. Supp. 421 (E.D. Va. 1989); Del Zio v. Presbyterian Hosp., No. 74 Civ. 3558 (CES), 1978 U.S. Dist. LEXIS 14450 (S.D.N.Y. Nov. 9, 1978).

[23]See, e.g., In re Marriage of Litowitz, 48 P.3d 261 (Wash. 2002); J.B. v. M.B., 783 A.2d 707 (N.J. 2001); A.Z. v. B.Z., 725 N.E.2d 1051 (Mass. 2000); Kass v. Kass, 696 N.E.2d 174 (N.Y. 1998); Davis v. Davis, 842 S.W.2d 588 (Tenn. 1992).

[24]See http://www.kentlaw.edu/islt/TABLEIII.htm (last visited March 24, 2005).

[25]See, e.g., Massachusetts, where a statute prohibits the use of embryos for experimental purposes. See Mass. Gen. Laws Ann. ch. 112, 12J (prohibiting experimentation on live fetus either before or after it is implanted in uterus).

[26]Forbes v. Woods, 71 F. Supp. 2d 1015 (1999); Lifchez v. Hartigan, 735 F. Supp. 1361 (1990).

[27]http://www.ncsl.org/programs/health/genetics/rt-shcl.htm.

[28]http://www.ncsl.org/programs/health/genetics/rt-shcl.htm.

[29]http://www.ncsl.org/programs/health/genetics/rt-shcl.htm.

[30]http://www.ncsl.org/programs/health/genetics/rt-shcl.htm.

from many aspects of this law and subject instead to new guidelines to be adopted by the newly created California Institute for Regenerative Medicine.

State laws on dispositional authority over embryos and on hES cell research are in flux and are largely untested in the courts. Investigators working with NT or hES cell lines are well advised to seek advice on the latest rules applicable in their states.

REGULATION OF hES CELL AND NT RESEARCH IN OTHER COUNTRIES

There is no international consensus yet on whether and how to pursue hES cell research. For example, in February 2005, a committee of the U.N. General Assembly abandoned attempts to craft a global treaty on NT research and satisfied itself with a plurality vote in favor of a nonbinding resolution calling for a ban on all forms of human cloning or genetics research that are contrary to "human dignity," a phrase left to the interpretation of member countries.[31] Thus, the regulation of hES cell research varies from country to country. In many cases, there is no law explicitly addressing such research. In some countries, such as Poland and Italy, the research is forbidden or substantially curtailed. In others, however, there seems to be a trend toward liberalization of the laws. France and Germany, for example, have taken steps to permit research on cell lines derived from surplus *in vitro* fertilization (IVF) blastocysts,[32] and Japan[33] and Sweden[34] have lifted restrictions on making blastocysts for research with NT.

Given the increasing frequency of international collaboration in hES cell research, it is important to monitor regulatory developments in other countries. As the guidelines recommended by this committee in Chapter 6 require that the provenance of hES cell lines be consistent with the ethical standards and procedures adopted here, understanding the points of similarity and difference between the guidelines and the rules in other countries will help investigators and the ESCRO committees proposed in Chapter 3 to manage collaboration.

Some countries place limitations on the importation of cell lines whose origins are inconsistent with their laws. Australia, for example, adopted the Research Involving Human Embryos Act in 2002 and the Human Cloning Act, which prohibits NT for reproductive or therapeutic purposes.[35] Of possible importance to U.S.

---

[31]Associated Press, U.N. Group Calls for Cloning Ban, Feb. 18, 2005.

[32]"Europe Sends Mixed Signals on Stem-Cell Work," Victoria Knight, *Wall Street Journal* Jan. 26 2005. Note that that German liberalization applies only to cell lines produced prior to 2002. See http://www.germany-info.org/relaunch/education/new/edu_stemcells.html.

[33]http://web2.innovationworld.net/biotechconnect/000312.html.

[34]http://www.geocities.com/giantfideli/art/CellNEWS_Sw_thera_cloning.html.

[35]Research Involving Human Embryos Act, 2002, No. 145, 2002, An Act to regulate certain activities involving the use of human embryos, and for related purposes (http://scaleplus.law.gov.au/html/comact/browse/TOCN.htm); Prohibition of Human Cloning Act 2002, No. 144, 2002, An Act to prohibit human cloning and other unacceptable practices associated with reproductive technology, and for related purposes (http://scaleplus.law.gov.au/html/comact/browse/TOCN.htm).

investigators seeking to collaborate with Australian centers, Australia forbids the importation of cloned, parthenogenetic, androgenetic, or chimeric embryos (a chimeric embryo is defined as one in which nonhuman cells have been introduced into a human embryo). It is also an offense to create a human embryo by any method other than fertilization and for any purpose other than for the treatment of infertility. So-called hybrid embryos are specifically forbidden and such entities are defined to include an animal egg into which the nucleus of a human cell has been introduced. Commercial trading in human eggs, sperm, or embryos is not allowed. Those bans are backed by criminal sanctions with prison terms of up to 15 years, depending on the offense.

Australia's law allows research to be performed on embryos remaining in excess of clinical need, and the consent requirements for donors are consistent with those outlined in this committee's recommendations (see Chapter 5). Research is subject to oversight by a new committee, the National Health and Medical Research Council Licensing Committee, which has the authority to review research programs, grant licenses, and maintain a database regarding the licenses granted. That committee also has the authority to inspect licensee facilities to ensure compliance with its licensing conditions.

The United Kingdom has adopted an approach that depends on a central licensing authority, called the Human Fertilisation and Embryology Authority (HFEA). The role of HFEA is to monitor and license clinics that carry out any of the established IVF or other assisted reproductive technology procedures and to regulate human embryo research and the storage of reproductive materials. As in the present committee's Recommendation 8 above, donors in the United Kingdom must give consent for use of their gametes or embryos in research. Egg and sperm donors are paid a nominal fee and reasonable expenses.[36]

HFEA will grant a license to make embryos for research only if the research program meets the purposes outlined in U.K. law. Allowable research purposes include increasing knowledge of genetic disorders, developing better contraceptive techniques, and advancing the treatment of infertility. As of early 2005, HFEA had granted 28 research licenses, including 10 related to hES cells and two related to parthenogenesis.[37] Two licenses were granted for work with NT blastocysts.[38]

The United Kingdom also has created a Stem Cell Bank, launched by the Medical Research Council in September 2002. The bank exists to establish fully characterized and quality-controlled cell lines (see Chapter 5 for a discussion on banking). The cell lines will be supplied to accredited scientific research teams and eventually to pharmaceutical companies to enable the development of broad-ranging cell therapies.[39]

---

[36]http://www.hfea.gov.uk/PressOffice/Archive/34673456).

[37]http://www.hfea.gov.uk/Research.

[38]See "British to Clone Human Embryos for Stem Cells," Rick Weiss, *Washington Post*, February 9, 2005; Page A02; see also http://www.hfea.gov.uk/PressOffice/Archive/1092233888.

[39]http://www.hfea.gov.uk/PressOffice/Backgroundpapers/Stemcellresearch.

Israel does not have a central licensing authority, but it does have well-developed guidelines emerging out of the work of the Bioethics Advisory Committee of the Israel Academy of Sciences and Humanities, and, because the Health Ministry delegates decisions regarding new genetic research involving human beings to the Helsinki Committee for Genetic Experiments on Human Subjects, it also has a centralized review process for hES cell research.[40] Consistent with the guidelines proposed in this report, the Israeli guidelines require informed consent from donors of surplus blastocysts. The guidelines state that best practices include mentioning research uses from the beginning of the IVF process and separating the medical team responsible for the IVF treatment and donation from the scientific teams involved in embryo research who receive the donation. As in the recommendations made in the next chapter, buying and selling of embryos is forbidden in Israel, but making new embryos solely for research, including blastocysts made by NT, is permissible. Research and possible applications must be justifiable in terms of the benefit that it offers humanity, and confidentiality and privacy of the donors should be respected. As in the recommendation proposed in Chapter 3 for purely *in vitro* work on hES cell lines, Israel allows such work to be conducted without further need for specific ethical authorization.

In June 2002, Singapore's Bioethics Advisory Committee released its report *Ethical, Legal and Social Issues in Human Stem Cell Research, Reproductive and Therapeutic Cloning*, in which it recommended that NT be permitted under centralized regulation. Consistent with the guidelines proposed here, the regulatory framework should require the informed voluntary consent of donors, prohibit the commerce and sale of donated materials, require strong scientific justification before making new embryos solely for research purposes, and stipulate that no one shall be under a duty to participate in any manner of research on human stem cells to which he or she has a conscientious objection. The report has been presented to the relevant ministries, and the government will decide on the recommendations later.[41]

Canada is still debating legislation to regulate assisted reproductive technologies and embryo research, but it operates under guidelines that incorporate both centralized and local review. Under the guidelines issued by the Canadian Institute for Health Research,[42] review and approval by the central Stem Cell Oversight Committee, by local research ethics boards (REBs), and, where appropriate, by animal care committees is required for all research involving the derivation, *in vitro* study, and clinical trial of hES cell lines. At any time, however, the local REB or animal care committee may refer an hES cell research proposal to the Stem Cell Oversight Committee for ethics review if it considers the research to be within the oversight committee's purview according to the above criteria. Such decisions by the

---

[40]http://www.academy.ac.il/bioethics/articles/embryonic_ibc_report.pdf.
[41]www.bioethics-singapore.org.
[42]http://www.cihr-irsc.gc.ca/e/15349.html.

REB or animal care committee are not subject to appeal. Like the guidelines recommended in this report, the Canadian guidelines require a medical rationale for the research, the informed consent of donors, protection of donors' privacy, and a prohibition on payment to donors (see Chapter 5). And like the current policy of the U.S. government (but unlike that of New Jersey or California), the Canadian guidelines prohibit public financial support for making embryos solely for research or of research in which hES cells are combined with a nonhuman embryo.[43]

CONCLUSION

Despite the lack of federal funding for most hES cell research underway in the United States, several sets of federal regulations govern various aspects of hES cell research—human subjects protections for oocyte and some blastocyst donors, medical privacy protections, laboratory and safety standards, animal welfare requirements, and rules governing the importation of biological materials or the transfer of medical data from other countries. In many other countries where hES cell research is permitted and publicly funded, its practice is regulated by statute or other government policy. Those regulations address matters such as whether embryos may be made solely for research purposes; whether they may be made using NT, parthenogenesis, or androgenesis; whether human hES cells may be combined with nonhuman materials; and whether facilities and researchers must be licensed before engaging in hES cell research.

As hES cell research in the United States increases, it is essential that institutions and investigators adhere to existing applicable regulatory requirements, and given the increasing frequency of international collaboration in hES cell research, it will be important to monitor regulatory developments in other countries. The ESCRO committees proposed in this report will be charged with ensuring that U.S. investigators follow standards and procedures consistent with current regulations and with the guidelines recommended in this report. Various jurisdictions differ in their mechanisms for oversight and review. As discussed in Chapter 3, the committee recommends both local review of hES cell research by an institutional ESCRO committee and the establishment of a national body to serve as a forum for considering new developments in the scientific, clinical, and public policy issues surrounding hES cell research and for periodic review of the relevant guidelines. The distinction between local review and oversight and national consideration of larger policy issues is in line with current U.S. practice in other fields. An analogy is the current use of local institutional IBCs to regulate recombinant DNA research and the RAC to consider policy issues related to gene therapy. The dual mechanism will fulfill oversight and monitoring functions equivalent to the various systems mandated by other countries.

---

[43]http://www.cihr-irsc.gc.ca/e/1487.html.

5

Recruiting Donors and Banking hES Cells

The emergence of assisted reproductive technology (ART) more than 20 years ago has enabled many couples to overcome fertility problems. Nationwide, 107,587 ART procedures were performed in 2001 at 385 medical centers in the United States and U.S. territories; they resulted in the birth of 40,687 infants from 29,344 pregnancies (Wright et al., 2004). Nationally, 75 percent of ART treatments used fresh, fertilized embryos from the patients' own oocytes; 14 percent used thawed embryos from the patients' oocytes; 8 percent used fresh, fertilized embryos from donor oocytes; and 3 percent used thawed embryos from donor oocytes. Thus, procedures can involve gametes from the couples themselves or from donors.

Various ART procedures result in the production of more embryos than are needed. Couples can choose to cryopreserve (freeze) and store these "extra" embryos for future attempts at establishing pregnancy. Embryos are often cryopreserved in *in vitro* fertilization (IVF) practices because transfer of more than three embryos per cycle increases risks for the mother and offspring and cryopreserved embryos offer fairly high pregnancy rates upon eventual transfer (Klock, 2004). Frozen embryos accumulate at a rate of about four per cycle. It is estimated that more than 400,000 embryos are stored in the United States (Hoffman et al., 2003), and there are nearly 16,000 embryos in storage in Canada (Baylis et al., 2003).

Once a couple decides to terminate their fertility treatment, for whatever reason, they have a number of options regarding the disposition of these embryos: they can donate them to another couple, they can make them available for quality assurance activities, they can donate them for research purposes, they can dispose of them, or they can store them indefinitely (Hoffman, et al., 2003). Many industrialized countries have developed laws or guidelines to govern the disposition of embryos. National regulations vary from eternal preservation to 5-year and 10-year preservation limits (Moutel et al., 2002; Grubb, 1996).

In addition to excess blastocysts, there might be excess gametes—oocytes and sperm that have been collected for IVF procedures from the couples themselves or from donors—that are no longer needed for reproductive purposes. Women not seeking infertility treatments might elect to donate oocytes for research purposes as an adjunct to a clinical intervention (such as oophorectomy) or as a straightforward altruistic donation specifically for research.

A number of studies have shown that some couples are willing to donate unneeded blastocysts for research purposes—as many as 25 percent in some studies (Bangsboll et al., 2004; Burton and Sanders, 2004; Klock, 2004; McMahon et al., 2003). The attitudes of couples who have undergone IVF range from almost parental concern for the embryos to regarding them as medical byproducts with little relationship to a couple's having a living child. Respondents positively disposed to donation commented on their desire not to waste blastocysts, a desire to help infertile couples, or a desire to advance scientific knowledge. Those with negative views commented on the embryo as a potential child and expressed concerns about a perceived lack of control over the type of research to be performed (McMahon et al. 2003).

Ethical principles dictate that potential donors of gametes or blastocysts for human embryonic stem cell (hES cell) research be able to make voluntary and informed choices about whether and how to donate their materials for research and that there be a clear option of "informed refusal," that is, the right to preclude any research use of embryos. Because of concerns about possible coercion or exploitation of potential donors and controversy regarding the moral status of embryos, it is important that precautions be taken in recruiting donors and ensuring their informed voluntary consent. Some of the protections offered through existing federal regulations can be adapted for application to hES cell research, such as adherence to principles of informed consent and a requirement that an Institutional Review Board (IRB) review the consent process. In addition, Food and Drug Administration (FDA) regulations should be considered for some types of research, specifically if there is a need to retain identifying information about the donors. That has implications for the consent process and for plans to protect confidentiality and privacy of information. Because of privacy concerns, certain provisions of the Health Insurance Portability and Accountability Act (HIPAA) might also apply. (Those regulatory requirements were discussed in Chapter 4.)

In this chapter, the committee makes specific detailed recommendations for IRB review of procurement (as recommended in the previous chapter); for the consent processes for obtaining somatic cells, gametes, and blastocysts for use in hES cell research; and for storing and maintaining cell lines once derived. Important safeguards must be in place to ensure that materials are collected ethically and that, once obtained, they are used for scientifically meritorious research (see also Chapters 2 and 3) with the confidentiality of donors protected.

REVIEW OF THE PROCUREMENT AND INFORMED CONSENT PROCESS

As discussed in Chapter 4, although the federal regulations governing human subjects research apply directly only to federally sponsored research or research conducted to secure FDA approval, many research institutions have implemented policies that require that all human subjects research conducted at the institution—regardless of the source of funding—abide by the federal requirements, primarily IRB review and the need for voluntary informed consent of subjects.

If an institution abides by the research regulations, it must invoke IRB review whenever human subjects research is conducted unless the research is exempt under the regulations. In addition, if hES cell lines obtained from donated materials are maintained with tracking codes, which might be required for research intended for clinical application, such research could transform donors into "research subjects" because study of the tissue could reveal information about them (unless the information was coded in such a way as to be unidentifiable by the investigator). Because FDA donor-suitability rules for transplants of cells or tissues from hES cell lines (discussed in Chapter 4) will probably require such tracking back to the donors, best practices suggest treating the donors as though they might be research subjects—that is, obtaining IRB review and approval of the consent process—to avoid problems later. In addition, even in the absence of tracking information, the process of donation could benefit from IRB experience in assessing the potential for inducements and risks and in reviewing the consent processes—all of which is relevant to the recruitment of donors of somatic cells, gametes, and blastocysts. As discussed in Chapter 4, this committee recommends that an IRB review the process by which material is obtained and that in all cases donors of cells, gametes, or blastocysts provide their informed consent. That requirement should extend to donors of gametes used in the IVF process.

Recommendation 13:
When donor gametes have been used in the *in vitro* fertilization process, resulting blastocysts may not be used for research without consent of all gamete donors.

The committee recognizes that this recommendation might eliminate from research some blastocysts that are in excess of clinical need, but that should not impose a major impediment to research, and the requirement for voluntary informed consent of all donors is an absolute prerequisite.

Thus, a researcher who wishes to obtain human oocytes or blastocysts for hES cell research must either request and obtain IRB review at his or her own institution (if one exists) to ensure that the informed consent provisions of the federal regulations at 45 CFR 46.116-117 and FDA regulations at 21 CFR 50.20-27 are followed or require that the fertility clinic have its own process for obtaining review from some other duly constituted IRB. The hES cell researcher should maintain a written record documenting the IRB review. IRB documentation should include an assurance of compliance with the relevant requirements in this report and relevant regulations and a copy of the consent form used for procurement purposes.

Ensuring that Donation Is Voluntary

Preceding sets of guidelines have emphasized the critical requirement of voluntary donation, including the explicit prohibition of monetary inducement or promise of therapeutic benefit. The original National Institutes of Health guidelines for hES cell research developed in 2000 stated "To ensure that the donation of human embryos in excess of the clinical need is voluntary, no inducements, monetary or otherwise, should have been offered for the donation of human embryos for research purposes. Fertility clinics and/or their affiliated laboratories should have implemented specific written policies and practices to ensure that no such inducements are made available." Likewise, the Canadian guidelines state "Neither the oocyte nor the sperm from which the embryos were created, nor the embryos themselves, were obtained through commercial transactions, including exchange for service." The European Commission and the U.K. Medical Research Council have instituted similar prohibitions. And the provisions of California's Proposition 71, passed in 2004, similarly prohibit payment to donors. Thus, there is virtual unanimity that to avoid any temptation for individuals to create extra embryos for research purposes, no payments should be offered for donation of residual embryos created for reproductive purposes in IVF programs. It is also agreed that there should be no added expense or burden to patients when residual blastocysts are donated and all storage costs for frozen blastocysts should be assumed by the investigators once donation has been confirmed.

The explanation of such unanimity might lie in the view that the treatment of the developing human embryo as an entity deserving of respect may be undermined by the introduction of a commercial motive into the solicitation or donation of fetal or embryonic tissue for research purposes. But although the potential for pressure is probably greatest when financial incentives are present, some nonfinancial incentives also should be avoided. For example, a donor's decisions should not be influenced by anticipated personal medical benefits or by concerns about the quality of later care. Any suggestion of personal benefit to a donor or to a person known to the donor should be avoided. (For obvious reasons, the use of nuclear transfer [NT] to develop hES cells for autologous transplantation requires that the recipient be specified.) Thus, a potential donor should be informed that there is no obligation to donate, that no personal benefit will accrue as a result of a decision to donate (except in cases of autologous transplantation), and that no penalty will result from a decision to refuse to donate. Similarly, people who elect to donate stored blastocysts for research should not be reimbursed for the costs of storage before the decision to donate, because this may be interpreted as an incentive to donate.

Recommendation 14:
To facilitate autonomous choice, decisions related to the production of em-bryos for infertility treatment should be free of the influence of investigators who propose to derive or use hES cells in research. Whenever it is practicable, the attending physician responsible for the infertility treatment and the investi-gator deriving or proposing to use hES cells should not be the same person.

Recommendation 15:
No cash or in kind payments may be provided for donating blastocysts in excess of clinical need for research purposes.

Recruiting and Paying Donors of Gametes for Research Purposes

Although there is widespread consensus that donors should not be paid for blastocysts they donate for research, there is less consensus about inducements for women to donate oocytes or men to donate sperm for research purposes. It is probably least problematic when women opt to donate oocytes for research in conjunction with a clinical procedure already scheduled (such as IVF or oophorec-tomy). It is most problematic in the case of oocyte donation solely for research purposes, because the invasiveness and risks of the procedure suggest that financial remuneration is most deserved, but at the same time there is a greater likelihood of enticing potential donors to do something that poses some risk to themselves. Of course, some women might wish to donate oocytes solely for research for nonfinan-cial motives; such a desire might exist among women who have family or friends affected by a particular disease that might be better understood or treated in the future if hES cells were used.

If the need for oocytes in hES cell research increases, it is possible that donations from clinical procedures or for nonfinancial motives may prove insufficient to meet the demand. In such cases—for example, for research involving NT or for research requiring blastocysts that have not been frozen—investigators might want to recruit oocyte donors. In the context of human subjects research, use of advertising to recruit subjects is not considered objectionable, but it is deemed worthy of review. In the context of clinical research, FDA considers direct advertising for study sub-jects to be the start of the informed consent process and subject selection; therefore, advertisements should be reviewed and approved by an IRB.

No matter how donors are recruited, the issue of whether they should be paid remains. Paying research subjects is "a common and long-standing practice in the United States" (Dickert et al., 2002; Anderson and Weijer, 2002), perhaps because of the need to provide incentives as part of recruitment and because moral principles of fairness and gratitude support providing payment to those who bear the burdens of research on behalf of society. But how much money gamete donors should receive and what they should receive payment for (for example, time, inconvenience, discomfort, or level of risk) are still contested because of fears that remuneration—or some level of remuneration—will undermine voluntary informed consent.

Although the consensus is that remuneration of participants in research should be just and fair, there is little agreement in theory or in practice about what constitutes just or fair payment. Moreover, federal regulations and guidance are relatively quiet on the subject, warning about "undue influence" without specifying what counts as undue. One difficulty is that "undue influence" depends on context. The level at which remuneration is set will influence the decisions of some more than others. A major ethical concern is that payments should not be so high as to create an undue influence or offer undue inducement that could compromise a prospective donor's evaluation of the risks or the voluntariness of her choices. That concern is greatest when studies involve significant risks. Other concerns are that payments should not be so low as to recruit disproportionately high numbers of economically disadvantaged persons and that they should compensate participants fairly for their contribution to research.

In its guidance on "Payment to Research Subjects," FDA notes that "financial incentives are often used when health benefits to subjects are remote or nonexistent. The amount and schedule of all payments should be presented to the IRB at the time of initial review. The IRB should review both the amount of payment and the proposed method and timing of disbursement to assure that neither are coercive or present undue influence" (21 CFR 50.20). In particular, the FDA guidance indicates that payment should be prorated for the time of participation in the study rather than extended to study completion, because the latter could compromise a participant's right to withdraw at any time.

Many argue that research subjects, or in this case gamete donors, should be paid for their time and inconvenience, as well as their direct expenses, but are concerned about providing payment for incurring risk, a practice that some ethicists would rule out altogether. However, attitudes may differ considerably when the risk is a minor and transient symptom or discomfort (such as sleepiness or dizziness) rather than a substantial harm. Some arguments for limiting payment to time and inconvenience reflect a belief that participation in research should be an altruistic act. It is almost certainly true, however, that the prospect of financial remuneration motivates many people to participate in research and that it is often a necessary and sometimes a sufficient condition for their participation.

Thus, although payments to volunteers in research studies can be characterized as compensation, honoraria, or inducements, it is widely agreed that volunteers should be reimbursed for direct expenses. Similarly, offering a small or token honorarium after participation is generally accepted. The consensus is less clear on whether volunteers should be paid for time and lost wages. Some consider that a form of compensation and there is disagreement about whether amounts should depend on income. The value placed on a person's time depends in part on the person's socioeconomic status, but there are concerns about using poverty as a justification for perpetuating differential payments.

Inducements are commonly provided for competent adult research subjects and some argue that oocyte donation should be treated in a similar fashion and that it is inappropriately paternalistic to prohibit competent women from making an informed choice. Others believe that the reproductive context makes this special and that payment should be prohibited. Underlying those principled concerns is a more pragmatic debate about whether (and how much) payment is needed to ensure a sufficient supply of oocytes for stem cell research.

Recommendation 16:
Women who undergo hormonal induction to generate oocytes specifically for research purposes (such as for nuclear transfer) should be reimbursed only for direct expenses incurred as a result of the procedure, as determined by an Institutional Review Board. No cash or in kind payments should be provided for donating oocytes for research purposes. Similarly, no payments should be made for donations of sperm for research purposes or of somatic cells for use in nuclear transfer.

This recommendation is based, in part, on the recognition that payments to oocyte donors raise concerns that might undermine public confidence in the responsible management of hES cell research. Following the recommendation will ensure consistency between procurement practices here and in other countries that have major hES cell research programs, thus facilitating international collaborations and the sharing of hES cell lines across national borders. It also ensures consistency with the limitations enacted in California in Proposition 71, facilitating collaboration between California investigators and those in the rest of the country.

The committee recognizes the strengths of all the arguments surrounding this issue. The recommendation should not be interpreted as a commentary on commercial IVF practices, but as a narrow policy position specifically with respect to hES cell research. Further, as with all the policies recommended by the committee, this policy should be regularly reviewed and reconsidered as the field matures and the experiences under other policies can be evaluated.

Finally, it is important to note that oocyte donation is not without risks. Oocyte donors undergoing ovulation induction have a small risk of severe ovarian hyperstimulation syndrome (OHSS). OHSS may affect 2-5 percent of women undergoing stimulation and can sometimes require hospital admission (Orvieto, 2005; ASRM, 2004a; Endo et al., 2002). Careful monitoring and adjustment of the medication regimen during the stimulation treatment can reduce the risk of OHSS. Risks posed by donation must be clearly articulated and understood by the prospective donor. In the United States—where insurance coverage varies and often does not cover research-related costs—the donor must be informed of whether and how much compensation is available if she is injured as a result of research. In general, compensation is not assured.

TIMING OF THE DECISION TO DONATE EXCESS BLASTOCYSTS

It is widely accepted that, whenever possible, donors' decisions to dispose of their blastocysts should be made separately from their decisions to donate them for research. Potential donors should be allowed to provide blastocysts for research only if they have decided to have those blastocysts discarded instead of donating them to another couple or storing them. If the decision to discard the blastocysts precedes the decision to donate them for research purposes, the research will determine only how their destruction occurs, not whether it occurs (NBAC, 1999a). The U.K. Medical Research Council guidelines emphasize the separation of tissue collection from the practice of research: "Those collecting embryos or adult cells/tissues, or involved in the process of fetal termination, and those responsible for the clinical care of the donor, should not knowingly be involved in research on those human tissues."

That separation may not always be possible, particularly because the couple may be informed of several options simultaneously at the outset of treatment for infertility or after its completion. Some infertility programs provide patients with multiple consent forms at the outset of treatment, forms that include options to donate to research, discard, or transfer any embryos that remain. When embryos are created for infertility treatment, couples are often asked to stipulate what should be done with frozen embryos in the event of future contingencies, such as death, divorce, or the inability of the clinic to contact them at a later date (ASRM, 2002). In addition, given growing public awareness about hES cell research, some couples might request at the outset of treatment that they be provided the opportunity to donate unneeded embryos to research. However, even if couples indicated at the outset of their clinical treatment that they chose to donate excess embryos for research, that decision must be confirmed before the embryos are thawed for research use (Lo et al., 2004).

Recommendation 17:
Consent for blastocyst donation should be obtained from each donor at the time of donation. Even people who have given prior indication of their intent to donate to research any blastocysts that remain after clinical care should nonetheless give informed consent at the time of donation. Donors should be informed that they retain the right to withdraw consent until the blastocysts are actually used in cell line derivation.

INFORMED CONSENT REQUIREMENTS

Prospective donors of blastocysts or gametes that remain after infertility treatment and donors of gametes for research should receive timely, relevant, and appropriate information to make informed and voluntary choices. Before considering the potential research use of the blastocysts, a prospective donor should have been presented with the option of storing the embryos, donating them to another woman or couple, donating them to research, or discarding them.

The current regulatory system specifies basic elements of information that must be provided to prospective participants during the informed consent process. In the context of donation for research, disclosure should ensure that potential donors understand the risks involved, if any. Donors should be told of all options concerning the care and disposition of their embryos, including freezing for later use, donation to others for reproductive use, research use, or discard without research use (Lo et al., 2004). To the extent possible, donors should be informed of the variety of future research uses before giving consent to donate blastocysts for research. Written informed consent must be obtained from all those who elect to donate blastocysts or gametes. Comprehensive information must be provided to all donors that is readily accessible and at a level that will enable an informed decision to be made.

Potential Discovery of Clinically Significant Information

If the identity of the donor is to be retained in a way that is ascertainable to the investigator, donors should be informed of the possibility that relevant clinical information might be discovered in the course of the research (for example, a genetic mutation conferring carrier status). There is ongoing debate about whether findings from research should be communicated to research subjects (donors would be considered subjects if identifiable information about them were known to researchers), either upon completion of a study or at some later date in time. This issue is relevant to all research, not just research involving hES cell lines. The obligation to report such findings to the donors depends in large part on the reliability of the findings and the significance of the information to human health.

MacKay has written that preliminary results do not yet constitute "information" since "until an initial finding is confirmed, there is no reliable information" to communicate to subjects, and that "even . . . confirmed findings may have some unforeseen limitations" (MacKay, 1984). McKay and others have argued that subjects should not be given information about their individual research results until the findings have been confirmed through the development of a reliable, accurate, and valid confirmatory test (MacKay, 1984; Fost and Farrell, 1989). On the other hand, those who believe that persons have the right to research results cite the principle of autonomy, which dictates that persons have a right to know what has been learned about them, and that therefore, interim results should be shared with subjects (Veatch, 1981).

Confusion about the appropriateness of returning individual research findings has increased as a result of HIPAA's Standards for Privacy of Individually Identifiable Health Information (the Privacy Rule; see Chapter 4). The Privacy Rule provides an individual the right of access to information about himself or herself, including personal research results obtained in the course of clinical care, with limited exceptions. The Privacy Rule not only gives patients a right to see their own records but also requires that patients be notified of their right to see such records. This regulatory requirement is most likely to lead to an increase in the number of persons who are aware of and exercise their right to request and receive research findings, all of which will have implications for the researcher. Investigators will have to be prepared to include, and IRBs to review, plans for how to respond to subjects' requests for disclosure of research findings. Clearly, in the clinical context it is the utility and validity of the information that should dictate a decision to recontact individuals. It is less clear whether an investigator, who has no therapeutic relationship with the person, has the same obligation.

Another important requirement must be considered in the decision to report research findings to subjects—the Clinical Laboratory Improvement Amendments of 1988 (CLIA). CLIA regulations do not permit the return of research results to patients or subjects if the tests were not conducted in a CLIA-approved laboratory. Thus, if a research laboratory is not CLIA-approved, it should not be reporting its results to subjects. In some circumstances, repeating the test in a CLIA-approved laboratory may be feasible and appropriate.

In any case, donors should be clearly informed in the consent process whether they will have the opportunity to receive individual results from the project. Whether it is appropriate to return the results will depend on several factors and should be subject to IRB review.

Recommendation 18:
In the context of donation of gametes or blastocysts for hES cell research, the informed consent process, should, at a minimum, provide the following information:

> a. **A statement that the blastocysts or gametes will be used to derive hES cells for research that may include research on human transplantation.**
> b. **A statement that the donation is made without any restriction or direction regarding who may be the recipient of transplants of the cells derived, except in the case of autologous donation.**
> c. **A statement as to whether the identities of the donors will be readily ascertainable to those who derive or work with the resulting hES cell lines.**
> d. **If the identities of the donors are retained (even if coded), a statement as to whether donors wish to be contacted in the future to receive information obtained through studies of the cell lines.**
> e. **An assurance that participants in research projects will follow applicable and appropriate best practices for donation, procurement, culture, and storage of cells and tissues to ensure, in particular, the traceability of stem cells. (Traceable information, however, must be secured to ensure confidentiality.)**
> f. **A statement that derived hES cells and/or cell lines might be kept for many years.**

g. A statement that the hES cells and/or cell lines might be used in research involving genetic manipulation of the cells or the mixing of human and nonhuman cells in animal models.

h. Disclosure of the possibility that the results of study of the hES cells may have commercial potential and a statement that the donor will not receive financial or any other benefits from any future commercial development;

i. A statement that the research is not intended to provide direct medical benefit to the donor(s) except in the case of autologous donation.

j. A statement that embryos will be destroyed in the process of deriving hES cells.

k. A statement that neither consenting nor refusing to donate embryos for research will affect the quality of any future care provided to potential donors.

l. A statement of the risks involved to the donor.

In addition, donors could be offered the option of agreeing to some forms of hES cell research but not others. For example, donors might agree to have their materials used for deriving new hES cell lines but might not want their materials used, for example, for NT. The consent process should fully explore whether donors have objections to any specific forms of research to ensure that their wishes are honored.

ADHERENCE TO STANDARDS OF CLINICAL CARE

Clinical facilities providing ART services have an obligation to protect the rights and safety of their patients and to behave in an ethical manner. Researchers must not pressure members of the fertility treatment team to generate more embryos than necessary for the optimum chance of reproductive success. An IVF clinic, or other third party responsible for obtaining consent and/or collecting materials should not be able to pay for or be paid for the material it obtains (apart from specifically defined, cost-based reimbursements). Placing such restrictions on paying those who obtain the embryos discourages the creation during routine infertility procedures of excess embryos that would later be used for research purposes.

Finally, no member of the medical or nursing staff should be under any duty to participate in providing donor information or securing donor consent for research use of gametes or blastocysts if he or she has a conscientious objection. However, this privilege does not extend to the appropriate clinical care of a donor or recipient.

Recommendation 19:
Consenting or refusing to donate gametes or embryos for research should not affect or alter in any way the quality of care provided to prospective donors. That is, clinical staff must provide appropriate care to patients without prejudice regarding their decisions about disposition of their embryos.

Recommendation 20:
Clinical personnel who have a conscientious objection to hES cell research should not be required to participate in providing donor information or securing donor consent for research use of gametes or blastocysts. That privilege should not extend to the care of a donor or recipient.

Recommendation 21:
Researchers may not ask members of the infertility treatment team to generate more oocytes than necessary for the optimal chance of reproductive success. An infertility clinic or other third party responsible for obtaining consent or collecting materials should not be able to pay for or be paid for the material obtained (except for specifically defined cost-based reimbursements and payments for professional services).

Restricting payment of those who obtain the embryos discourages the production of excess embryos during routine infertility procedures for later use in research. Other measures can be taken to ensure that conflicts of interest are appropriately managed. For example, the embryologist in the ART program who makes the determination that an oocyte has failed to fertilize or develop sufficiently for implantation should not be a member of the hES research team.

BANKING AND DISTRIBUTION OF CELL LINES

Once donated materials are obtained from couples or individuals, several additional standards should be applied to the storage, maintenance, and distribution of cell lines for research use. People and institutions responsible for these activities must maintain the highest ethical, legal, and scientific standards (Brivanlou et al., 2003). Cell lines might be stored at several institutions as part of individual research collections or might be deposited in more central repositories or banks. Developing standardized practices for obtaining, screening, processing, validating, and storing cell lines, and distributing them to users will provide confidence to researchers and the public that the materials are of high quality and of optimal use to researchers.

Several models exist for the banking of human biological materials. The most relevant is the U.K. Stem Cell Bank, which was established to provide researchers with an independent national stem cell resource:[1]

The Cell Bank will offer a vital resource to support the advance of research in this exciting area. At the same time it will develop important safeguards, by ensuring that cell lines which could ultimately provide the basis for clinical treatment are appropriately characterized and also handled and stored under conditions that are

---

[1]http://www.nibsc.ac.uk/divisions/cbi/stemcell.html.

properly controlled. This will not only provide high quality starting materials to facilitate the development of stem cell therapy, but, in providing a centralized resource for researchers, should also reduce the use of surplus embryos for the development of stem cell lines by individual teams.

One of the conditions of the U.K. bank's establishment was the development of an extensive code of practice for its operations (Medical Research Council, 2004). In addition, it has a clear system of governance, which involves a steering committee for policy, a management committee, and a user and clinical liaison committee.

Tissue-banking policies and practices in connection with a wide array of human cells, tissues, and organs have been established by several public and private entities in the United States, including the National Cancer Institute,[2] the National Heart, Lung and Blood Institute,[3] and private entities, such as Coriell[4] and the American Type Culture Collection.[5] In addition, the U.S. Office for Human Research Protections (OHRP) has issued two guidance documents: *Issues to Consider in Research Use of Stored Data or Tissues*[6] and *Guidance on Research Involving Coded Private Information or Biological Specimens.*[7]

The guidelines developed by those groups and the U.K. Stem Cell Bank generally adhere to key ethical principles that focus on the need for consent of donors and a system for monitoring adherence to ethical, legal, and scientific requirements. For example, a common requirement is that any identifiable tissue (including coded tissue) that is collected requires IRB review at the site of collection and informed consent of the subject. In addition, most require that, when possible, the informed consent process include information about the repository and the conditions under which materials will be shared. Other policies address the need to protect the privacy of donors. Several models exist for protecting subjects whose specimens are used for research, including the honest-broker model, in which a tissue bank trustee ensures strict control of information flows associated with research that uses banked tissues (see the model developed by OHRP[8]).

Procedurally, it is common practice that there be a clear policy and system for evaluating requests for samples to see whether each request is consistent with the conditions for sharing samples and with the original informed consent.

At the repository management level, there typically are requirements for safety, security, and risk assessments; validation of submitted material; culturing and ex-

---

[2]www.cancerdiagnosis.nci.nih.gov/specimenes/brochure.html; www.cancerdiagnosis.nci.nih.gov/specimens/legal.html.

[3]www.nhlbi.nih.gov/funding/policies/repos-gl.htm.

[4]http://locus.umdnj.edu/.

[5]http://www.atcc.org/.

[6]http://www.hhs.gov/ohrp/humansubjects/guidance/reposit.htm.

[7]http://www.hhs.gov/ohrp/humansubjects/guidance/cdebiol.pdf.

[8]http://www.hhs.gov/ohrp/humansubjects/guidance/reposit.htm.

pansion of cell line; process control; packaging, labeling, and distribution; and documentation and data management. Those requirements, in addition to routine quality assurance and control, will be as critical in hES cell research as in any other field that uses human materials. As hES cell research advances, it will be increasingly important for institutions that are obtaining, storing, and using cell lines to have confidence in the value of stored cells—that is, that they were obtained ethically and with the informed consent of donors, that they are well characterized and screened for safety, and that the conditions under which they are maintained and stored meet the highest scientific standards.

Recommendation 22:
Institutions that are banking or plan to bank hES cell lines should establish uniform guidelines to ensure that donors of material give informed consent through a process approved by an Institutional Review Board, and that meticulous records are maintained about all aspects of cell culture. Uniform tracking systems and common guidelines for distribution of cells should be established.

Recommendation 23:
Any facility engaged in obtaining and storing hES cell lines should consider the following standards:

(a) Creation of a committee for policy and oversight purposes and creation of clear and standardized protocols for banking and withdrawals.
(b) Documentation requirements for investigators and sites that deposit cell lines, including
    (i)   A copy of the donor consent form.
    (ii)   Proof of Institutional Review Board approval of the procurement process.
    (iii)   Available medical information on the donors, including results of infectious-disease screening.
    (iv)   Available clinical, observational, or diagnostic information about the donor(s).
    (v)   Critical information about culture conditions (such as media, cell passage, and safety information).
    (vi)   Available cell line characterization (such as karyotype and genetic markers).
A repository has the right of refusal if prior culture conditions or other items do not meet its standards.

(c) A secure system for protecting the privacy of donors when materials retain codes or identifiable information, including but not limited to

(i)   A schema for maintaining confidentiality (such as a coding system).
(ii)   A system for a secure audit trail from primary cell lines to those submitted to the repository.
(iii)   A policy governing whether and how to deliver clinically significant information back to donors.

(d) The following standard practices:
(i)   Assignment of a unique identifier to each sample.
(ii)   A process for characterizing cell lines.
(iii)   A process for expanding, maintaining, and storing cell lines.
(iv)   A system for quality assurance and control.
(v)   A website that contains scientific descriptions and data related to the cell lines available.
(vi)   A procedure for reviewing applications for cell lines.
(vii)   A process for tracking disbursed cell lines and recording their status when shipped (such as number of passages).
(viii) A system for auditing compliance.
(ix)   A schedule of charges.
(x)   A statement of intellectual property policies.
(xi)   When appropriate, creation of a clear Material Transfer Agreement or user agreement.
(xii)   A liability statement.
(xiii) A system for disposal of material.

(e) Clear criteria for distribution of cell lines, including but not limited to evidence of approval of the research by an Embryonic Stem Cell Research Oversight committee or equivalent body at the recipient institution.

The committee also notes and commends recent efforts at the federal level by the National Institutes of Health[9] to encourage the sharing and dissemination of important research resources. Restricted availability of unique research resources, such as hES cell lines, upon which further studies are dependent, can impede the advancement of research. To the extent possible, the committee encourages practices that make cell lines readily available in a timely fashion to the research community for further research, development, and application.

---

[9]See NIH's Policy on Sharing of Model Organisms for Biomedical Research at http://grants.nih.gov/grants/guide/notice-files/NOT-OD-04-042.html.

SUMMARY

Individuals and couples who voluntarily and with full information donate somatic cells, gametes, or blastocysts for hES research must be assured that the research will be meritorious and that all possible efforts will be made by those with responsibility for handling, storing, and using resulting cell lines to protect donor confidentiality. The combination of IRB review of the procurement process and a process of fully informed consent before donation will contribute to the ethical conduct of the research. Once hES cells are derived, the proper banking and distribution of hES cell lines will maintain the covenant between donor and scientific community.

6

National Academies Guidelines for Research on Human Embryonic Stem Cells

1.0 Introduction
2.0 Establishment of an Institutional Embryonic Stem Cell Research Oversight Committee
3.0 Procurement of Gametes, Blastocysts or Cells for hES Generation
4.0 Derivation of hES Cell Lines
5.0 Banking and Distribution of hES Cell Lines
6.0 Research Use of hES Cell Lines
7.0 International Collaboration
8.0 Conclusion

1.0 INTRODUCTION

In this chapter we collect all the recommendations made throughout the report and translate them into a series of formal guidelines. These guidelines focus on the derivation, procurement, banking, and use of human embryonic stem (hES) cell lines. They provide an oversight process that will help to ensure that research with hES cells is conducted in a responsible and ethically sensitive manner and in compliance with all regulatory requirements pertaining to biomedical research in general. The National Academies are issuing these guidelines for the use of the scientific community, including researchers in university, industry, or other private-sector research organizations.

1.1(a) What These Guidelines Cover

These guidelines cover all derivation of hES cell lines and all research that uses hES cells derived from

(1) Blastocysts made for reproductive purposes and later obtained for research from *in vitro* fertilization (IVF) clinics.
(2) Blastocysts made specifically for research using IVF.
(3) Somatic cell nuclear transfer (NT) into oocytes.

The guidelines do not cover research that uses nonhuman stem cells.

Many, but not all, of the guidelines and concerns addressed in this report are common to other areas of human stem cell research, such as

(1) Research that uses human adult stem cells.
(2) Research that uses fetal stem cells or embryonic germ cells derived from fetal tissue; such research is covered by federal statutory restrictions at 42 U.S.C. 289g-2(a) and federal regulations at 45 CFR 46.210.

Institutions and investigators conducting research using such materials should consider which individual provisions of these guidelines are relevant to their research.

1.1(b) Reproductive Uses of NT

These guidelines also do not apply to reproductive uses of nuclear transfer (NT), which are addressed in the 2002 report *Scientific and Medical Aspects of Human Reproductive Cloning*, in which the National Academies recommended that "Human reproductive cloning should not now be practiced. It is dangerous and likely to fail." Although these guidelines do not specifically address human reproductive cloning, it continues to be the view of the National Academies that research aimed at the reproductive cloning of a human being should not be conducted at this time.

1.2 Categories of hES Cell Research

These guidelines specify categories of research that:

(a) Are permissible after currently mandated reviews and proper notification of the relevant research institution.
(b) Are permissible after additional review by an Embryonic Stem Cell Research Oversight (ESCRO) committee, as described in Section 2.0 of the guidelines.
(c) Should not be conducted at this time.

Because of the sensitive nature of some aspects of hES cell research, these guidelines in many instances set a higher standard than is required by laws or regulations with which institutions and individuals already must comply.

1.2(a) hES Cell Research Permissible after Currently Mandated Reviews

Purely *in vitro* hES cell research that uses previously derived hES cell lines is permissible provided that the ESCRO committee or equivalent body designated by the investigator's institution (see Section 2.0), receives documentation of: i) the provenance of the cell lines; ii) appropriate informed consent in their derivation; and iii) evidence of compliance with any required review by an Institutional Review Board (IRB), Institutional Animal Care and Use Committee (IACUC), or Institutional Biosafety Committee (IBC), or other mandated review.

1.2(b) hES Cell Research Permissible Only after Additional Review and Approval

(1) Generation of new lines of hES cells by whatever means.

(2) Research involving the introduction of hES cells into nonhuman animals at any stage of embryonic, fetal, or postnatal development; particular attention should be paid to the probable pattern and effects of differentiation and integration of the human cells into the nonhuman animal tissues.

(3) Research in which the identity of the donors of blastocysts, gametes, or somatic cells from which the hES cells were derived is readily ascertainable or might become known to the investigator.

1.2(c) hES Cell Research That Should Not Be Permitted at This Time

The following types of research should not be conducted at this time:

(1) Research involving *in vitro* culture of any intact human embryo, regardless of derivation method, for longer than 14 days or until formation of the primitive streak begins, whichever occurs first.

(2) Research in which hES cells are introduced into nonhuman primate blastocysts or in which any embryonic stem cells are introduced into human blastocysts.

In addition:

(3) No animal into which hES cells have been introduced at any stage of development should be allowed to breed.

1.3 Obligations of Investigators and Institutions

All scientific investigators and their institutions, regardless of their field, bear the ultimate responsibility for ensuring that they conduct themselves in accordance with professional standards and with integrity. In particular, people whose research involves hES cells should work closely with oversight bodies, demonstrate respect for the autonomy and privacy of those who donate gametes, blastocysts, or somatic cells and be sensitive to public concerns about research that involves human embryos.

2.0 ESTABLISHMENT OF AN INSTITUTIONAL EMBRYONIC STEM CELL RESEARCH OVERSIGHT COMMITTEE

To provide oversight of all issues related to derivation and use of hES cell lines and to facilitate education of investigators involved in hES cell research, each institution involved in hES cell research should establish an Embryonic Stem Cell Research Oversight (ESCRO) committee. The committee should include representatives of the public and persons with expertise in developmental biology, stem cell research, molecular biology, assisted reproduction, and ethical and legal issues in hES cell research. It must have suitable scientific, medical, and ethical expertise to conduct its own review and should have the resources needed to coordinate the management of the various other reviews required for a particular protocol. A pre-existing committee could serve the functions of the ESCRO committee provided that it has the recommended expertise and representation to perform the various roles described in this report. For example, an institution might elect to constitute an ESCRO committee from among some members of an IRB. But the ESCRO committee should not be a subcommittee of the IRB, as its responsibilities extend beyond human subject protections. Furthermore, much hES cell research does not require IRB review. The ESCRO committee should:

(1) Provide oversight over all issues related to derivation and use of hES cell lines.
(2) Review and approve the scientific merit of research protocols.
(3) Review compliance of all in-house hES cell research with all relevant regulations and these guidelines.
(4) Maintain registries of hES cell research conducted at the institution and hES cell lines derived or imported by institutional investigators.
(5) Facilitate education of investigators involved in hES cell research.

3.0 PROCUREMENT OF GAMETES, BLASTOCYSTS, OR CELLS FOR hES GENERATION

3.1. An IRB, as described in federal regulations at 45 CFR 46.107, should review the procurement of all gametes, blastocysts, or somatic cells for the purpose of generating new hES cell lines, including the procurement of blastocysts in excess of clinical need from infertility clinics, blastocysts made through IVF specifically for research purposes, and oocytes, sperm, and somatic cells donated for development of hES cell lines derived through NT or by parthenogenesis or androgenesis.

3.2. Consent for donation should be obtained from each donor at the time of donation. Even people who have given prior indication of their intent to donate to research any blastocysts that remain after clinical care should nonetheless give informed consent at the time of donation. Donors should be informed that they retain the right to withdraw consent until the blastocysts are actually used in cell line derivation.

3.3. When donor gametes have been used in the IVF process, resulting blastocysts may not be used for research without consent of all gamete donors.

3.4a. No payments, cash or in kind, may be provided for donating blastocysts in excess of clinical need for research purposes. People who elect to donate stored blastocysts for research should not be reimbursed for the costs of storage prior to the decision to donate.

3.4b. Women who undergo hormonal induction to generate oocytes specifically for research purposes (such as for NT) should be reimbursed only for direct expenses incurred as a result of the procedure, as determined by an IRB. No payments, cash or in kind, should be provided for donating oocytes for research purposes. Similarly, no payments should be made for donations of sperm for research purposes or of somatic cells for use in NT.

3.5. To facilitate autonomous choice, decisions related to the creation of embryos for infertility treatment should be free of the influence of investigators who propose to derive or use hES cells in research. Whenever it is practicable, the attending physician responsible for the infertility treatment and the investigator deriving or proposing to use hES cells should not be the same person.

3.6. In the context of donation of gametes or blastocysts for hES cell research, the informed consent process, should, at a minimum, provide the following information.

(a) A statement that the blastocysts or gametes will be used to derive hES cells for research that may include research on human transplantation.

(b) A statement that the donation is made without any restriction or direction regarding who may be the recipient of transplants of the cells derived, except in the case of autologous donation.

(c) A statement as to whether the identities of the donors will be readily ascertainable to those who derive or work with the resulting hES cell lines.

(d) If the identities of the donors are retained (even if coded), a statement as to whether donors wish to be contacted in the future to receive information obtained through studies of the cell lines.

(e) An assurance that participants in research projects will follow applicable and appropriate best practices for donation, procurement, culture, and storage of cells and tissues to ensure, in particular, the traceability of stem cells. (Traceable information, however, must be secured to ensure confidentiality.)

(f) A statement that derived hES cells and/or cell lines might be kept for many years.

(g) A statement that the hES cells and/or cell lines might be used in research involving genetic manipulation of the cells or the mixing of human and nonhuman cells in animal models.

(h) Disclosure of the possibility that the results of study of the hES cells may have commercial potential and a statement that the donor will not receive financial or any other benefits from any future commercial development.

(i) A statement that the research is not intended to provide direct medical benefit to the donor(s) except in the case of autologous donation.

(j) A statement that embryos will be destroyed in the process of deriving hES cells.

(k) A statement that neither consenting nor refusing to donate embryos for research will affect the quality of any future care provided to potential donors.

(l) A statement of the risks involved to the donor.

In addition, donors could be offered the option of agreeing to some forms of hES cell research but not others. For example, donors might agree to have their materials used for deriving new hES cell lines but might not want their materials used, for example, for NT. The consent process should fully explore whether donors have objections to any specific forms of research to ensure that their wishes are honored.

3.7. Clinical personnel who have a conscientious objection to hES cell research should not be required to participate in providing donor information or securing donor consent for research use of gametes or blastocysts. That privilege should not extend to the care of a donor or recipient.

3.8. Researchers may not ask members of the infertility treatment team to generate more oocytes than necessary for the optimal chance of reproductive success. An infertility clinic or other third party responsible for obtaining consent or collecting materials should not be able to pay for or be paid for the material obtained (except for specifically defined cost-based reimbursements and payments for professional services).

4.0 DERIVATION OF hES CELL LINES

4.1. Requests to the ESCRO committee for permission to attempt derivation of new hES cell lines from donated embryos or blastocysts must include evidence of IRB approval of the procurement process (see Section 3.0 above).

4.2. The scientific rationale for the need to generate new hES cell lines, by whatever means, must be clearly presented, and the basis for the numbers of embryos and blastocysts needed should be justified.

4.3. Research teams should demonstrate appropriate expertise or training in derivation or culture of either human or nonhuman ES cells before permission to derive new lines is given.

4.4. When NT experiments involving either human or nonhuman oocytes are proposed as a route to generation of ES cells, the protocol must have a strong scientific rationale. Proposals that include studies to find alternatives to donated oocytes in this research should be encouraged.

4.5. Neither blastocysts made using NT (whether produced with human or nonhuman oocytes) nor parthenogenetic or androgenetic human embryos may be transferred to a human or nonhuman uterus or cultured as intact embryos *in vitro* for longer than 14 days or until formation of the primitive streak, whichever occurs first.

4.6. Investigators must document how they will characterize, validate, store, and distribute any new hES cell lines and how they will maintain the confidentiality of any coded or identifiable information associated with the lines (see Section 5.0 below).

5.0 BANKING AND DISTRIBUTION OF hES CELL LINES

There are several models for the banking of human biological materials, including hES cells. The most relevant is the U.K. Stem Cell Bank. The guidelines developed by this and other groups generally adhere to key ethical principles that focus on the need for consent of donors and a system for monitoring adherence to ethical, legal, and scientific requirements. As hES cell research advances, it will be increasingly important for institutions that are obtaining, storing, and using cell lines to have confidence in the value of stored cells—that is, that they were obtained ethically and with the informed consent of donors, that they are well characterized and screened for safety, and that the conditions under which they are maintained and stored meet the highest scientific standards. Institutions engaged in hES research should seek mechanisms for establishing central repositories for hES cell lines—through partnerships or augmentation of existing quality research cell line repositories and should adhere to high ethical, legal, and scientific standards. At a minimum, an institutional registry of stem cell lines should be maintained.

5.1 Institutions that are banking or plan to bank hES cell lines should establish uniform guidelines to ensure that donors of material give informed consent through a process approved by an IRB and that meticulous records are maintained about all aspects of cell culture. Uniform tracking systems and common guidelines for distribution of cells should be established.

5.2 Any facility engaged in obtaining and storing hES cell lines should consider the following standards:

(a) Creation of a committee for policy and oversight purposes and creation of clear and standardized protocols for banking and withdrawals.

(b) Documentation requirements for investigators and sites that deposit cell lines, including
(i) A copy of the donor consent form.
(ii) Proof of Institutional Review Board approval of the procurement process.
(iii) Available medical information on the donors, including results of infectious-disease screening.
(iv) Available clinical, observational, or diagnostic information about the donor(s).
(v) Critical information about culture conditions (such as media, cell passage, and safety information).
(vii)Available cell line characterization (such as karyotype and genetic markers).
A repository has the right of refusal if prior culture conditions or other items do not meet its standards.

(c) A secure system for protecting the privacy of donors when materials retain codes or identifiable information, including but not limited to
(i) A schema for maintaining confidentiality (such as a coding system).
(ii) A system for a secure audit trail from primary cell lines to those submitted to the repository.
(iii) A policy governing whether and how to deliver clinically significant information back to donors.

(d) The following standard practices:
(i)   Assignment of a unique identifier to each sample.
(ii)   A process for characterizing cell lines.
(iii)   A process for expanding, maintaining, and storing cell lines.
(iv)   A system for quality assurance and control.
(v)   A website that contains scientific descriptions and data related to the cell lines available.
(vi)   A procedure for reviewing applications for cell lines.
(vii) A process for tracking disbursed cell lines and recording their status when shipped (such as number of passages).
(viii) A system for auditing compliance.

(ix)   A schedule of charges.

(x)   A statement of intellectual property policies.

(xi)   When appropriate, creation of a clear Material Transfer Agreement or user agreement.

(xii)   A liability statement.

(xiii) A system for disposal of material.

(e)   Clear criteria for distribution of cell lines, including but not limited to evidence of approval of the research by an Embryonic Stem Cell Research Oversight committee or equivalent body at the recipient institution.

6.0   RESEARCH USE OF hES CELL LINES

Once hES cell lines have been derived, investigators and institutions, through ESCRO committees and other relevant committees (such as an IACUC, an IBC, or a radiation safety committee) should monitor their use in research.

6.1 Institutions should require documentation of the provenance of all hES cell lines, whether the cells were imported into the institution or generated locally. Notice to the institution should include evidence of IRB-approval of the procurement process and of adherence to basic ethical and legal principles of procurement. In the case of lines imported from another institution, documentation that these criteria were met at the time of derivation will suffice.

6.2. *In vitro* experiments involving the use of already derived and coded hES cell lines will not need review beyond the notification required in Section 6.1.

6.3. Each institution should maintain a registry of its investigators who are conducting hES cell research and ensure that all registered users are kept up to date with changes in guidelines and regulations regarding the use of hES cells.

6.4. All protocols involving the combination of hES cells with nonhuman embryos, fetuses, or adult animals must be submitted to the local IACUC for review of animal welfare issues and to the ESCRO committee for consideration of the consequences of the human contributions to the resulting chimeras. (See also Section 1.2(c)(3) concerning breeding of chimeras.)

6.5. Transplantation of differentiated derivatives of hES cells or even hES cells themselves into adult animals will not require extensive ESCRO committee review. If there is a possibility that the human cells could contribute in a major organized way to the brain of the recipient animal, however, the scientific justification for the experiments must be strong, and proof of principle using nonhuman (preferably primate) cells, is desirable.

6.6. Experiments in which hES cells, their derivatives, or other pluripotent cells are introduced into nonhuman fetuses and allowed to develop into adult chimeras need more careful consideration because the extent of human contribution to the resulting animal may be higher. Consideration of any major functional contributions to the brain should be a main focus of review. (See also Section 1.2(c)(3) concerning breeding of chimeras.)

6.7. Introduction of hES cells into nonhuman mammalian blastocysts should be considered only under circumstances in which no other experiment can provide the information needed. (See also Sections 1.2(c)(2) and 1.2(c)(3) concerning restrictions on breeding of chimeras and production of chimeras with nonhuman primate blastocysts.)

6.8 Research use of existing hES cells does not require IRB review unless the research involves introduction of the hES cells or their derivatives into patients or the possibility that the identity of the donors of the blastocysts, gametes, or somatic cells is readily ascertainable or might become known to the investigator.

7.0 INTERNATIONAL COLLABORATION

If a U.S.-based investigator collaborates with an investigator in another country, the ESCRO committee may determine that the procedures prescribed by the foreign institution afford protections consistent with these guidelines, and the ESCRO committee may approve the substitution of some of or all of the foreign procedures for its own.

8.0 CONCLUSION

The substantial public support for hES cell research and the growing trend by many nonfederal funding agencies and state legislatures to support this field requires a set of guidelines to provide a framework for hES cell research. In the absence of the oversight that would come with unrestricted federal funding of this research, these guidelines will offer reassurance to the public and to Congress that the scientific community is attentive to ethical concerns and is capable of self-regulation while moving forward with this important research.

To help ensure that these guidelines are taken seriously, stakeholders in hES cell research—sponsors, funding sources, research institutions, relevant oversight committees, professional societies, and scientific journals, as well as investigators—should develop policies and practices that are consistent with the principles inherent in these guidelines. Funding agencies, professional societies, journals, and institutional review panels can provide valuable community pressure and impose appropriate sanctions to ensure compliance. For example, ESCRO committees and IRBs should require evidence of compliance when protocols are reviewed for renewal, funding agencies should assess compliance when reviewing applications for support, and journals should require that evidence of compliance accompanies publication of results.

As individual states and private entities move into hES cell research, it will be important to initiate a national effort to provide a formal context in which the complex moral and oversight questions associated with this work can be addressed on a continuing basis. Both the state of hES cell research and clinical practice and public policy surrounding these topics are in a state of flux and are likely to be so for several years. Therefore, the committee believes that a national body should be established to assess periodically the adequacy of the policies and guidelines proposed in this document and to provide a forum for a continuing discussion of issues involved in hES cell research. New policies and standards may be appropriate for issues that cannot now be foreseen. The organization that sponsors this body should be politically independent and without conflicts of interest, should be respected in the lay and scientific communities, and able to call on suitable expertise to support this effort.

References

Allen, N. D., Barton, S. C., Hilton, K., Norris, M. L., and Surani, M. A. 1994. A functional analysis of imprinting in parthenogenetic embryonic stem cells. Development. 120:1473-1482.

Amit, M., Carpenter, M. K., Inokuma, M. S., Chiu, C. P., Harris, C. P., Waknitz, M. A., Itskovitz-Eldor, J., and Thomson, J. A. 2000. Clonally derived human embryonic stem cell lines maintain pluripotency and proliferative potential for prolonged periods of culture. Develomental Biology. 227:271-278.

Anderson J. A., and Weijer C. 2002. The research subject as wage earner. Theoretical Medicine and Bioethics. 23(4-5):359-376.

American Society for Reproductive Medicine (ASRM). Ethics Committee. 2000. Financial incentives in recruitment of oocyte donors. Fertility and Sterility. 74(2):216-220.

ASRM. Ethics Committee. 2002. Donating spare embryos for embryonic stem-cell research. Fertility and Sterility. 78(5):957-960.

ASRM. Ethics Committee. 2004a. Ovarian hyperstimulation syndrome. Fertility and Sterility. 82(Supplement 2):S81-86.

ASRM. Ethics Committee. 2004b. Donating spare embryos for embryonic stem-cell research. Fertility and Sterility. 82(Supplement 2):S224-S227.

Assady, S., Maor, G., Amit, M., Itskovitz-Eldor, J., Skorecki, K. L., and Tzukerman, M. 2001. Insulin production by human embryonic stem cells. Diabetes. 50:1691-1697.

Bangsboll S., Pinborg A., Yding Andersen C., and Nyboe Andersen A. 2004. Patients' attitudes towards donation of surplus cryopreserved embryos for treatment or research. Human Reproduction. 19(10):2415-2419.

Baylis F., Beagan B., Johnston J., and Ram N. 2003. Cryopreserved human embryos in Canada and their availability for research. Journal of Obstetrics and Gynaecology Canada. 25(12):1026-1031.

Bioethics Advisory Committee of Singapore. 2002. Ethical, Legal and Social Issues in Human Stem Cell Research, Reproductive and Therapeutic Cloning. Released June 21.

Bongso, A., Fong, C. Y., Ng, S. C., and Ratnam, S. 1994. Isolation and culture of inner cell mass cells from human blastocysts. Human Reproduction. 9:2110-2117.

Brivanlou, A. H., Gage, F. H., Jaenisch, R., Jessell, T., Melton, D., and Rossant, J. 2003. Setting Standards for Human Embryonic Stem Cells. Science. 300:913-916.

Burton P. J., and Sanders K. 2004. Patient attitudes to donation of embryos for research in Western Australia. The Medical Journal of Australia. 180(11):559-561.

Campbell, K. H., McWhir, J., Ritchie, W. A., and Wilmut, I. 1996. Sheep cloned by nuclear transfer from a cultured cell line. Nature. 380:64-66.

Carpenter, M. K., and Bhatia, M. 2004. Characterization of Human Embryonic Stem Cells, Vol. 1 (Amsterdam, Elsevier).

Chadwick, K., Wang, L., Li, L., Menendez, P., Murdoch, B., Rouleau, A., and Bhatia, M. 2003. Cytokines and BMP-4 promote hematopoietic differentiation of human embryonic stem cells. Blood. 102:906-915.

Chen, Y., He, Z. X., Liu, A., Wang, K., Mao, W. W., Chu, J. X., Lu, Y., Fang, Z. F., Shi, Y. T., Yang, Q. Z., Chen, D. Y., Wang, M. K., Li, J. S., Huang, S. L., Kong, X. Y., Shi, Y. Z., Wang, Z. Q., Xia, J. H., Long, Z. G., Xue, Z. G., Ding, W. X., and Sheng, H., Z.. 2003. Embryonic stem cells generated by nuclear transfer of human somatic nuclei into rabbit oocytes. Cell Research. 13:251-263.

Cibelli, J. B., Grant, K. A., Champman, K. B., Lanza, R. P., Vrana, K. E., Cunniff, K., Worst, T., Green, H., Walker, S., Gutin, P., Vilner, L., Tabar, V., Dominko, T., Kane, J., Wettstein, P., Studer, L., and West, M. 2002. Parthenogenetic stem cells in nonhuman primates. Science. 295:819.

Congregation of the Doctrine of the Faith. 1987. Instruction on Respect for Human Life in Its Origin and on the Dignity of Procreation. Vatican City.

Daheron, L., Opitz, S. L., Zaehres, H., Lensch, W. M., Andrews, P. W., Itskovitz-Eldor, J., and Daley, G. Q. 2004. LIF/STAT3 signaling fails to maintain self-renewal of human embryonic stem cells. Stem Cells. 22:770-778.

Delhaise, F., Bralion, V., Schuurbiers, N., and Dessy, F. 1996. Establishment of an embryonic stem cell line from 8-cell stage mouse embryos. European Journal of Morphology. 34:237-243.

Department of Health, Education, and Welfare (DHEW). Ethics Advisory Board (EAB). 1979. Report and Conclusions: HEW Support of Research Involving Human In Vitro Fertilization and Embryo Transfer. Washington, D.C.: U.S. Government Printing Office.

Dickert N., Emanuel E., and Grady C. 2002. Paying research subjects: an analysis of current policies. Annals of Internal Medicine. 136(5):368-373.

Doetschman, T., Gregg, R. G., Maeda, N., Hooper, M. L., Melton, D. W., Thompson, S., and Smithies, O. 1987. Targeted correction of a mutant HPRT gene in mouse embryonic stem cells. Nature. 330:576-578.

Edwards, R. G., ed. 2004. History of Embryo Stem Cells (Amsterdam, Elsevier).

Eiges, R., Schuldiner, M., Drukker, M., Yanuka, O., Itskovitz-Eldor, J., and Benvenisty, N. 2001. Establishment of human embryonic stem cell-transfected clones carrying a marker for undifferentiated cells. Current Biology. 11:514-518.

Endo, T., Honnma, H., Hayashi, T., Chida, M., Yamazaki, K., Kitajima, Y., Azumaguchi, A., Kamiya, H., and Kudo, R. 2002. Continuation of GnRH agonist administration for 1 week, after hCG injection, prevents ovarian hyperstimulation syndrome following elective cryopreservation of all pronucleate embryos. Human Reproduction. 17(10):2548-2551.

Evans, M. J., and Kaufman, M. H. 1981. Establishment in culture of pluripotential cells from mouse embryos. Nature. 292:154-156.

Fost, N., and Farrell, P.M. 1989. A prospective randomized trial of early diagnosis and treatment of cystic fibrosis: A unique ethical dilemma. Clinical Research. 37:495–500.

Gardner, R. L. 2004. Pluripotent Stem Cells from Vertebrate Embryos: Present Perspective and Future Challenges, Vol. 1 (Amsterdam, Elsevier).

Goldstein, R. S., Drukker, M., Reubinoff, B. E., and Benvenisty, N. 2002. Integration and differentiation of human embryonic stem cells transplanted to the chick embryo. Developmental Dynamics. 225:80-86.

Gropp, M., Itsykson, P., Singer, O., Ben-Hur, T., Reinhartz, E., Galun, E., and Reubinoff, B. E. 2003. Stable genetic modification of human embryonic stem cells by lentiviral vectors. Molecular Therapy. 7:281-287.

Grubb, A. 1996. The Human Fertilisation and Embryology Act (Statutory Storage Period for Embryos) Regulations 1996 (S.I. 1996 No. 375). Medical Law Review. 4(2):211-215.

Hoffman, D. I., Zellman, G. L., Fair, C. C., Mayer, J. F., Zeitz, J. G., Gibbons, W. E., and Turner, T. G. 2003. Cryopreserved embryos in the United States and their availability for research. Fertility and Sterility. 79(5):1063-1069.

Hubner, K., Fuhrmann, G., Christenson, L. K., Kehler, J., Reinbold, R., De La Fuente, R., Wood, J., Strauss, J. F., 3rd, Boiani, M., and Scholer, H. R. 2003. Derivation of oocytes from mouse embryonic stem cells. Science. 300:1251-1256.

Hurlbut. 2004. PCB; http://www.bioethics.gov/transcripts/dec04/dec3full.html.

Hwang, W. S., Ryu, Y. J., Park, J. H., Park, E. S., Lee, E. G., Koo, J. M., Jeon, H. Y., Lee, B. C., Kang, S. K., Kim, S. J., Ahn, C., Hwang, J. H., Ky Young Park, K. Y., Cibelli, J. B., and Moon, S. Y. 2004. Evidence of a pluripotent human embryonic stem cell line derived from a cloned blastocyst. Science. 303:1669-1674.

Itskovitz-Eldor, J., Schuldiner, M., Karsenti, D., Eden, A., Yanuka, O., Amit, M., Soreq, H., and Benvenisty, N. 2000. Differentiation of human embryonic stem cells into embryoid bodies compromising the three embryonic germ layers. Molecular Medicine. 6:88-95.

Jaenisch, Rudolph. 2004. Human Cloning — The Science and Ethics of Nuclear Transplantation. The New England Journal of Medicine. 351(27):2787-2791.

Kaufman, D. S., Hanson, E. T., Lewis, R. L., Auerbach, R., and Thomson, J. A. 2001. Hematopoietic colony-forming cells derived from human embryonic stem cells. PNAS. 98:10716-10721.

Kaufman, M. H., Robertson, E. J., Handyside, A. H., and Evans, M. J. 1983. Establishment of pluripotential cell lines from haploid mouse embryos. J. Embryol. Exp. Morphol. 73:249-261.

Kawase, E., Yamazaki, Y., Yagi, T., Yanagimachi, R., and Pedersen, R. A. 2000. Mouse embryonic stem (ES) cell lines established from neuronal cell-derived cloned blastocysts. Genesis. 28:156-163.

Kehat, I., Kenyagin-Karsenti, D., Snir, M., Segev, H., Amit, M., Gepstein, A., Livne, E., Binah, O., Itskovitz-Eldor, J., and Gepstein, L. 2001. Human embryonic stem cells can differentiate into myocytes with structural and functional properties of cardiomyocytes. Journal of Clinical Investigation. 108:407-414.

Klimanskaya, I., and McMahon, J. 2004. Isolation and Maintenance of Human ES Cells: Detailed Procedures and Alternatives, Vol 1 (Amsterdam, Elsevier).

Klock, S. C. 2004. Embryo disposition: the forgotten "child" of in vitro fertilization. International Journal of Fertility and Womens Medicine. 49(1):19-23.

Klug, M. G., Soonpaa, M. H., Koh, G. Y., and Field, L. J. 1996. Genetically selected cardiomyocytes from differentiating embryonic stem cells form stable intracardiac grafts. Journal of Clinical Investigation. 98:216-224.

Kyba, M., Perlingeiro, R. C., and Daley, G. Q. 2002. HoxB4 confers definitive lymphoid-myeloid engraftment potential on embryonic stem cell and yolk sac hematopoietic progenitors. Cell. 109:29-37.

Landry, D. W., and Zucker, H. A. 2004. Embryonic death and the creation of human embryonic stem cells. The Journal of Clinical Investigation.114:1184-1186.

Lanza, R., Gearhart, J., Hogan, B., Melton, D. W., Pedersen, R., Thomson, J., and West, M. 2004. Handbook of Stem Cells, Vol. 1 (Amsterdam, Elsevier).

Levenberg, S., Golub, J. S., Amit, M., Itskovitz-Eldor, J., and Langer, R. 2002. Endothelial cells derived from human embryonic stem cells. PNAS. 99:4391-4396.

Lo, B., Chou, V., Cedars, M. I., Gates, E., Taylor, R. N., Wagner, R. M., Wolf, L., Yamamoto, K. R. 2004. Informed consent in human oocyte, embryo, and embryonic stem cell research. Fertility and Sterility. 83(3):559-563.

Ma, Y., Ramezani, A., Lewis, R., Hawley, R. G., and Thomson, J. A. 2003. High-level sustained transgene expression in human embryonic stem cells using lentiviral vectors. Stem Cells. 21:111-117.

MacKay, C. R. 1984. Ethical issues in research design and conduct: developing a test to detect carriers of Huntington's disease. IRB. 6(4):1–5.

Mann, J. R., Gadi, I., Harbison, M. L., Abbondanzo, S. J. and Stewart, C. L. 1990. Androgenetic mouse embryonic stem cells are pluripotent and cause skeletal defects in chimeras: implications for genetic imprinting. Cell. 62:251-60.

Martin, G. R. 1981. Isolation of a pluripotent cell line from early mouse embryos cultured in medium conditioned by teratocarcinoma stem cells. PNAS. 78: 7634-7638.

Martin, M. J., Muotri, A., Gage, F., and Varki, A. 2005. Human embryonic stem cells express an imunogenic nonhuman sialic acid. Nature Medicine. 11(2):228-232.

Matsui, Y., Zsebo, K., and Hogan, B. L. M. 1992. Derivation of pluripotential embryonic stem cells from murine primordial germ cells in culture. Cell. 70:841-847.

McMahon C. A., Gibson F. L., Leslie G. I., Saunders D. M., Porter K. A., and Tennant C. C. 2003. Embryo donation for medical research: attitudes and concerns of potential donors. Human Reproduction. 18(4):871-877.

Melton, D. A., Daley, G. Q., and Jennings, C. G. 2004. Altered nuclear transfer in stem-cell research—a flawed proposal. New England Journal of Medicine. 351:2791-2792.

Medical Research Council (MRC). 2004. Code of Practice for the Use of Human Stem Cell Lines (interim). United Kingdom. [Online]. Available: http://www.mrc.ac.uk/index/public-interest/public-consultation/public-stem-cell-consultation.htm.

Moutel, G., Gregg, E., Meningaud, J. P., and Herve, C. 2002. Developments in the storage of embryos in France and the limitations of the laws of bioethics. Analysis of procedures in 17 storage centres and the destiny of stored embryos. Medicine and Law. 21(3):587-604.

Mummery, C., Ward, D., van den Brink, C. E., Bird, S. D., Doevendans, P. A., Opthof, T., Brutel de la Riviere, A., Tertoolen, L., van der Heyden, M., and Pera, M. 2002. Cardiomyocyte differentiation of mouse and human embryonic stem cells. J. Anat. 200:233-242.

Munsie, M. J., Michalska, A. E., O'Brien, C. M., Trounson, A. O., Pera, M. F., and Mountford, P. S. 2000. Isolation of pluripotent embryonic stem cells from reprogrammed adult mouse somatic cell nuclei. Current Biology 10:989-992.

Nagy, A., Gocza, E., Diaz, E. M., Prideaux, V. R., Ivanyi, E., Markkula, M., and Rossant, J. 1990. Embryonic stem cells alone are able to support fetal development in the mouse. Development. 110:815-821.

Nagy, A., Rossant, J., Nagy, R., Abramow-Newerly, W., and Roder, J. C. 1993. Derivation of completely cell culture-derived mice from early-passage embryonic stem cells. PNAS. 90:8424-8428.

National Bioethics Advisory Commission (NBAC). 1997. Cloning Human Beings. 2 vols. Rockville, Md.: U.S. Government Printing Office.

NBAC. 1999a. Ethical Issues in Human Stem Cell Research. Volume I. Report and Recommendations. Rockville, Md.: U.S. Government Printing Office.

NBAC. 1999b. Ethical Issues in Human Stem Cell Research. Volume III. Religious Prespectives. Rockville, Md.: U.S. Government Printing Office.

National Commission for the Protection of Human Subjects of Biomedical and Behavioral Research. 1975. Research on the Fetus: Report and Recommendations. Washington, D.C.: U.S. Government Printing Office.

NIH (National Institutes of Health). Human Embryo Research Panel. 1994. *Report of the Human Embryo Research Panel.* 2 volumes. Bethesda, M.D.

NIH). Office of the Director (OD). 1999. "Fact Sheet on Stem Cell Research." Bethesda, MD.

National Research Council (NRC). 2002a. Stem Cells and the Future of Regenerative Medicine. Washington, D.C.: National Academy Press.

NRC. 2002b. Scientific and Medical Aspects of Human Reproductive Cloning. Washington, D.C.: National Academy Press.

Nisbet, M. C. 2004. Public Opinion about stem cell research and human cloning. Public Opinion Quarterly 68(1):131-154.

O'Brien, M. J., Pendola, J. K., and Eppig, J. J. 2003. A revised protocol for in vitro development of mouse oocytes from primordial follicles dramatically improves their developmental competence. Biology of Reproduction. 68:682-1686.

Office of the White House Press Secretary, Statement by the President, December 2, 1994.

Orvieto, R. 2005. Can we eliminate severe ovarian hyperstimulation syndrome? Human Reproduction. 20(2):20-322.

Pera, M. F., and Trounson, A. O. 2004. Human embryonic stem cells: prospects for development. Development. 131:5515-5525.

Pfeifer, A., Ikawa, M., Dayn, Y., and Verma, I. M. 2002. Transgenesis by lentiviral vectors: lack of gene silencing in mammalian embryonic stem cells and preimplantation embryos. PNAS. 99:2140-2145.

President's Council on Bioethics. 2002. Human Cloning and Human Dignity: An Ethical Inquiry. Washington, D.C.

Resnick, J. L., Bixler, L. S., Cheng, L., and Donovan, P. J. 1992. Long-term proliferation of mouse primordial germ cells in culture. Nature. 359:550-552.

Reubinoff, B. E., Pera, M. F., Fong, C. Y., Trounson, A., and Bongso, A. 2000. Embryonic stem cell lines from human blastocysts: somatic differentiation in vitro. Nat. Biotechnol. 18:399-404.

Reubinoff, B. E., Itsykson, P., Turetsky, T., Pera, M. F., Reinhartz, E., Itzik, A., and Ben-Hur, T. 2001. Neural progenitors from human embryonic stem cells. Nature Biotechnology. 19:1134-1140.

Ridcout, W. M., 3rd, Hochedlinger, K., Kyba, M., Daley, G. Q., and Jaenisch, R. 2002. Correction of a genetic defect by nuclear transplantation and combined cell and gene therapy. Cell. 109:17-27.

Robert, J. S., and Baylis F. 2003. Crossing species boundaries. American Journal of Bioethics. 3(3):1-13.

Shamblott, M. J., Axelman, J., Wang, S., Bugg, E. M., Littlefield, J. W., Donovan, P. J., Blumenthal, P. D., Huggins, G. R., and Gearhart, J. D. 1998. Derivation of pluripotent stem cells from cultured human primordial germ cells. PNAS. 95:13726-13731.

Smith, A. G., Heath, J. K., Donaldson, D. D., Wong, G. G., Moreau, J., Stahl, M., and Rogers, D. 1988. Inhibition of pluripotential embryonic stem cell differentiation by purified polypeptides. Nature. 336:688-690.

Stewart, C. L. 1993. Production of Chimeras between Embryonic Stem Cells and Embryos, Vol. 225 (San Diego, Academic Press).

Szabo, P., and Mann, J. R. 1994. Expression and methylation of imprinted genes during in vitro differentiation of mouse parthenogenetic and androgenetic embryonic stem cell lines. Development. 120:1651-1660.

Thomas, K. R., and Capecchi, M. R. 1987. Site-directed mutagenesis by gene targeting in mouse embryo-derived stem cells. Cell. 51:503-512.

Thomson, J. A., Itskovitz-Eldor, J., Shapiro, S. S., Waknitz, M. A., Swiergiel, J. J., Marshall, V. S., and Jones, J. M. 1998. Embryonic stem cell lines derived from human blastocysts. Science. 282:1145-1147.

U.S. Congress, Office of Technology Assessment. 1988. Infertility: Medical and Social Choices. OTA-BA-358. Washington, D.C.: U.S. Government Printing Office.

Veatch, R. M. 1981. A Theory of Medical Ethics. New York: Basic Books.

Verlinsky, Y., Strelchenko, N., Kukharenko, V., Rechitsky, S., Veriinsky, O., Galat, V., and Kuliev, A. 2005. Human embryonic stem cell lines with genetic disorders. Reproductive BioMedicine Online. 10(I):105-110.

Wade, N. 1998. Researchers claim embryonic cell mix of human and cow. NY Times. Nov 12:A1, A26.

Wagers, A. J., and Weissman, I. L. 2004. Plasticity of adult stem cells. Cell. 116(5):639-648.

Wakayama, T., Tabar, V., Rodriguez, I., Perry, A. C., Studer, L., and Mombaerts, P. 2001. Differentiation of embryonic stem cell lines generated from adult somatic cells by nuclear transfer. Science. 292:740-743.

Walters, L. 2004. Human embryonic stem cell research: an intercultural perspective. Kennedy Institute of Ethics Journal. 14(1):3-38.

Wichterle, H., Lieberam, I., Porter, J. A., and Jessell, T. M. 2002. Directed differentiation of embryonic stem cells into motor neurons. Cell. 110(3):385-97.

Wiles, M. V. 1993. Embryonic Stem Cell Differentiation in Vitro, Vol. 225 (San Diego, Academic Press).

Williams, R. L., Hilton, D. J., Pease, S., Willson, T. A., Stewart, C. L., Gearing, D. P., Wagner, E. F., Metcalf, D., Nicola, N. A., and Gough, N. M. 1988. Myeloid leukaemia inhibitory factor maintains the developmental potential of embryonic stem cells. Nature. 336:684-687.

Windom, R.E. 1988. Memorandum to James B. Wyngaarden, March 22, 1988. Report of the Human Fetal Tissue Transplantation Research Panel. Vol. 2, A3. Bethesda, Md.: NIH.

Wright, V. C., Schieve, L.A., Reynolds, M. A., Jeng, G., and Kissin, D. 2004. Assisted reproductive technology surveillance—United States, 2001. Morbidity and Mortality Weekly Report. April 30: 1-20.

Xu, R. H., Chen, X., Li, D. S., Li, R., Addicks, G. C., Glennon, C., Zwaka, T. P., and Thomson, J. A. 2002. BMP4 initiates human embryonic stem cell differentiation to trophoblast. Nature Biotechnology. 20:1261-1264.

Xu, R. H., Peck, R. M., Li, D. S., Feng, X., Ludwig, T., and Thomson, J. A. 2005. Basic FGF and suppression of BMP signaling sustain undifferentiated proliferation of human ES cells. Nature Methods. 2(3):185-190

Zhang, S. C., Wernig, M., Duncan, I. D., Brustle, O., and Thomson, J. A. 2001. In vitro differentiation of transplantable neural precursors from human embryonic stem cells. Nature Biotechnology. 19:1129-1133.

Zwaka, T. P., and Thomson, J. A. 2003. Homologous recombination in human embryonic stem cells. Nature Biotechnology. 21:319-321.

Glossary

Adult stem cell—An undifferentiated cell found in a differentiated tissue that can renew itself and (with limitations) differentiate to yield the specialized cell types of the tissue from which it originated.

Androgenesis—Development in which the embryo contains only paternal chromosomes.

Autologous transplant—Transplanted tissue derived from the intended recipient of the transplant. Such a transplant helps to avoid complications of immune rejection.

Blastocoel—The cavity in the center of a blastocyst.

Blastocyst—A preimplantation embryo of 50–250 cells depending on age. The blastocyst consists of a sphere made up of an outer layer of cells (the trophectoderm), a fluid-filled cavity (the blastocoel), and a cluster of cells on the interior (the inner cell mass).

Blastomere—A single cell from a morula or early blastocyst, before the differentiation into trophectoderm and inner cell mass.

Bone marrow—The soft, living tissue that fills most bone cavities and contains hematopoietic stem cells, from which all red and white blood cells evolve. The bone marrow also contains mesenchymal stem cells from which a number of cell types arise, including chondrocytes, which produce cartilage, and fibroblasts, which produce connective tissue.

Chimera—An organism composed of cells derived from at least two genetically different cell types. The cells could be from the same or separate species.

Differentiation—The process whereby an unspecialized early embryonic cell acquires the features of a specialized cell, such as a heart, liver, or muscle cell.

DNA—Deoxyribonucleic acid, a chemical found primarily in the nucleus of cells. DNA carries the instructions for making all the structures and materials the body needs to function.

Ectoderm—The outermost of the three primitive germ layers of the embryo; it gives rise to skin, nerves, and brain.

Egg cylinder—An asymmetric embryonic structure that helps to determine the body plan of the mouse.

Electroporation— Method of introducing DNA into a cell.

Embryo—An animal in the early stages of growth and differentiation that are characterized by cleavage, laying down of fundamental tissues, and the formation of primitive organs and organ systems; especially the developing human individual from the time of implantation to the end of the eighth week after conception, after which stage it becomes known as a fetus.*

Embryoid bodies (EBs)—Clumps of cellular structures that arise when embryonic stem cells are cultured. Embryoid bodies contain tissue from all three germ layers: endoderm, mesoderm, and ectoderm. Embryoid bodies are not part of normal development and occur only in vitro.

Embryonic disk—A group of cells derived from the inner cell mass of the blastocyst, which later develops into an embryo. The disk consists of three germ layers known as the endoderm, mesoderm, and ectoderm.

Embryonic germ (EG) cells—Cells found in a specific part of the embryo or fetus called the gonadal ridge that normally develop into mature gametes. The germ cells differentiate into the gametes (oocytes or sperm).

Embryonic stem (ES) cells—Primitive (undifferentiated) cells derived from the early embryo that have the potential to become a wide variety of specialized cell types.

Endoderm—Innermost of the three primitive germ layers of the embryo; it later gives rise to the lungs, liver, and digestive organs.

Enucleated cell—A cell whose nucleus has been removed.

Epidermis—The outer cell layers of the skin.

---

* http://www.nlm.nih.gov/medlineplus/mplusdictionary.html. In common parlance, "embryo" is used more loosely and variably to refer to all stages of development from fertilization until some ill-defined stage when it is called a fetus. There are strictly defined scientific terms such as "zygote," "morula," and "blastocyst" that refer to specific stages of preimplantation development (see Chapter 2). In this report, we have used the more precise scientific terms where relevant but have used the term "embryo" where more precision seemed likely to confuse rather than clarify.

Epigenetic— Refers to modifications in gene expression that are controlled by heritable but potentially reversible changes in DNA methylation or chromatin structure without involving alteration of the DNA sequence.

Epithelium—Layers of cells in various organs, such as the epidermis of the skin or the lining of the gut. These cells serve the general functions of protection, absorption, and secretion, and play a specialized role in moving substances through tissue layers. Their ability to regenerate is excellent; the cells of an epithelium may replace themselves as frequently as every 24 hours from the pools of specialized stem cells.

Feeder cell layer—Cells that are used in culture to maintain pluripotent stem cells. Feeder cells usually consist of mouse embryonic fibroblasts.

Fertilization—The process whereby male and female gametes unite to form a zygote (fertilized egg).

Fibroblasts—Cells from many organs that give rise to connective tissue.

Gamete—A mature male or female germ cell, that is, sperm or oocyte, respectively.

Gastrulation—The procedure by which an animal embryo at an early stage of development produces the three primary germ layers: ectoderm, mesoderm, and endoderm.

Gene—A functional unit of heredity that is a segment of DNA located in a specific site on a chromosome. A gene usually directs the formation of an enzyme or other protein.

Gene targeting— A procedure used to produce a mutation in a specific gene.

Genital ridge—Anatomic site in the early fetus where primordial germ cells are formed.

Genome—The complete genetic material of an organism.

Genotype— Genetic constitution of an individual.

Germ cell—A sperm or egg or a cell that can become a sperm or egg. All other body cells are called somatic cells.

Germ layer—In early development, the embryo differentiates into three distinct germ layers (ectoderm, endoderm, and mesoderm), each of which gives rise to different parts of the developing organism.

Ger line—The cell lineage from which the oocyte and sperm are derived.

Gonadal ridge—Anatomic site in the early fetus where primordial germ cells (PGCs) are formed.

Gonads—The sex glands—testis and ovary.

Hematopoietic—Blood-forming.

Hematopoietic stem cell (HSC)—A stem cell from which all red and white blood cells evolve and that may be isolated from bone marrow or umbilical cord blood for use in transplants.

Hepatocyte—Liver cell.

Heterologous—From genetically different individuals.

hES cell—Human embryonic stem cell; a type of pluripotent stem cell.

Histocompatibility antigens—Glycoproteins on the surface membranes of cells that enable the body's immune system to recognize a cell as native or foreign and that are determined by the major histocompatibility complex.

Homologous recombination—Recombining of two like DNA molecules, a process by which gene targeting produces a mutation in a specific gene.

Hybrid— An organism that results from a cross between gametes of two different genotypes.

Immune system cells—White blood cells, or leukocytes, that originate in the bone marrow. They include antigen-presenting cells, such as dendritic cells, T and B lymphocytes, macrophages, and neutrophils, among many others.

Immunodeficient mice—Genetically altered mice used in transplantation experiments because they usually do not reject transplanted tissue.

Immunogenic—Related to or producing an immune response.

Immunosuppressive— Suppressing a natural immune response.

Implantation—The process in which a blastocyst implants into the uterine wall, where a placenta forms to nurture the growing fetus.

Inner cell mass—The cluster of cells inside the blastocyst that give rise to the embryonic disk of the later embryo and, ultimately, the fetus.

Interspecific—Between species.

In utero—In the uterus.

In vitro—Literally, "in glass," in a laboratory dish or test tube; in an artificial environment.

In vitro **fertilization (IVF)**—An assisted reproductive technique in which fertilization is accomplished outside the body.

In vivo—In the living subject; in a natural environment.

Karyotype—The full set of chromosomes of a cell arranged with respect to size, shape, and number.

Leukemia inhibitory factor (LIF)—A growth factor necessary for maintaining mouse embryonic stem cells in a proliferative, undifferentiated state.

Mesenchymal stem cells—Stem cells found in bone marrow and elsewhere from which a number of cell types can arise, including chondrocytes, which produce cartilage, and fibroblasts, which produce connective tissue.

Mesoderm—The middle layer of the embryonic disk, which consists of a group of cells derived from the inner cell mass of the blastocyst; it is formed at gastrulation and is the precursor to bone, muscle, and connective tissue.

Morula—A solid mass of 16–32 cells that resembles a mulberry and results from the cleavage (cell division without growth) of a zygote (fertilized egg).

Mouse embryonic fibroblast (MEF)—Cells used as feeder cells in culturing pluripotent stem cells.

Neural stem cell (NSC)—A stem cell found in adult neural tissue that can give rise to neurons, astrocytes, and oligodendrocytes.

Nuclear transfer (NT)—Replacing the nucleus of one cell with the nucleus of another cell.

Oocyte—Developing egg; usually a large and immobile cell.

Ovariectomy— Surgical removal of an ovary.

Parthenogenesis—Development in which the embryo contains only maternal chromosomes.

Passage—A round of cell growth and proliferation in culture.

Phenotype—Visible properties of an organism produced by interaction of genotype and environment.

Placenta—The oval or discoid spongy structure in the uterus from which the fetus derives its nourishment and oxygen.

Pluripotent cell—A cell that has the capability of developing into cells of all germ layers (endoderm, ectoderm, and mesoderm).

Precursor cells—In fetal or adult tissues, partly differentiated cells that divide and give rise to differentiated cells. Also known as progenitor cells.

Preimplantation genetic diagnosis (PGD)—A procedure applied to IVF embryos to determine which ones carry deleterious mutations predisposing to hereditary diseases.

Primary germ layers—The three initial embryonic germ layers—endoderm, mesoderm, and ectoderm—from which all other somatic tissue types develop.

Primordial germ cell—A cell appearing during early development that is a precursor to a germ cell.

Primitive streak—The initial band of cells from which the embryo begins to develop. The primitive streak establishes and reveals the embryo's head-tail and left-right orientations.

Pseudopregnant—Refers to a female primed with hormones to accept a blastocyst for implantation.

Somatic cells—Any cell of a plant or animal other than a germ cell or germ cell precursor.

Somatic cell nuclear transfer (SCNT)—The transfer of a cell nucleus from a somatic cell into an egg (oocyte) whose nucleus has been removed.

Stem cell—A cell that has the ability to divide for indefinite periods in vivo or in culture and to give rise to specialized cells.

Teratoma—A tumor composed of tissues from the three embryonic germ layers. Usually found in ovary or testis. Produced experimentally in animals by injecting pluripotent stem cells to determine the stem cells' abilities to differentiate into various types of tissues.

Tissue culture—Growth of tissue *in vitro* on an artificial medium for experimental research.

Transfection—A method by which experimental DNA may be put into a cultured cell.

Transgene—A gene that has been incorporated into a cell or organism and passed on to successive generations.

Transplantation—Removal of tissue from one part of the body or from one individual and its implantation or insertion into another, especially by surgery.

Trophectoderm—The outer layer of the developing blastocyst that will ultimately form the embryonic side of the placenta.

Trophoblast—The extraembryonic tissue responsible for negotiating implantation, developing into the placenta, and controlling the exchange of oxygen and metabolites between mother and embryo.

Undifferentiated—Not having changed to become a specialized cell type.

Xenograft or xenotransplant—A graft or transplant of cells, tissues, or organs taken from a donor of one species and grafted into a recipient of another species.

Zygote—A cell formed by the union of male and female germ cells (sperm and egg, respectively).

Abbreviations

ART	assisted reproductive technology
ASRM	American Society for Reproductive Medicine
CFR	Code of Federal Regulations
CGTP	current good tissue practices
CLIA	Clinical Laboratoy Improvement Amendments
DHEW	Department of Health, Education, and Welfare
DHHS	Department of Health and Human Services
EAB	Ethics Advisory Board
ES cell	embryonic stem cell
ESCRO	Embryonic Stem Cell Research Oversight
FDA	Food and Drug Administration
FDCA	Food, Drug, and Cosmetic Act
GLP	good laboratory practice
HCT/Ps	human cells, tissues, and cellular and tissue-based products
HERP	Human Embryo Research Panel
hEG cells	human embryonic germ cells
hES cells	human embryonic stem cells
HFEA	Human Fertilisation and Embryology Authority (United Kingdom)

HIPAA	Health Insurance Portability and Accountability Act
IACUC	Institutional Animal Care and Use Committee
IBC	Institutional Biosafety Committee
IDE	investigational device exemption
IND	investigational new drug
IRB	Institutional Review Board
IVF	*in vitro* fertilization
LIF	leukemia inhibitory factor
mES	mouse embryonic stem cells
NAS	National Academy of Sciences
NBAC	National Bioethics Advisory Commission
NIH	National Institutes of Health
NRC	National Research Council
NT	nuclear transfer
OHRP	Office for Human Research Protections
OHSS	ovarian hyperstimulation syndrome
PCB	President's Council on Bioethics
PGD	preimplantation genetic diagnosis
PHI	personal health information
PHS	Public Health Service
P.L.	Public law
RAC	Recombinant DNA Advisory Committee
rDNA	recombinant DNA
REB	Research Ethics Board (Canada)
SCNT	somatic cell nuclear transfer
USC	United States Code

Appendix A

Compilation of Recommendations

RECOMMENDATIONS FROM CHAPTER 3

Recommendation 1:
To provide local oversight of all issues related to derivation and research use of hES cell lines and to facilitate education of investigators involved in hES cell research, all institutions conducting hES cell research should establish an Embryonic Stem Cell Research Oversight (ESCRO) committee. The committee should include representatives of the public and persons with expertise in developmental biology, stem cell research, molecular biology, assisted reproduction, and ethical and legal issues in hES cell research. The ESCRO committee would not substitute for an Institutional Review Board but rather would provide an additional level of review and scrutiny warranted by the complex issues raised by hES cell research. The committee would also serve to review basic hES cell research using preexisting anonymous cell lines that does not require consideration by an Institutional Review Board.

Recommendation 2:
Through its Embryonic Stem Cell Research Oversight (ESCRO) committee, each research institution should ensure that the provenance of hES cells is documented. Documentation should include evidence that the procurement process was approved by an Institutional Review Board to ensure adherence to the basic ethical and legal principles of informed consent and protection of confidentiality.

Recommendation 3:
Embryonic Stem Cell Research Oversight (ESCRO) committees or their equivalents should divide research proposals into three categories in setting limits on research and determining the requisite level of oversight:

(a) Research that is permissible after notification of the research institution's ESCRO committee and completion of the reviews mandated by current requirements. Purely *in vitro* hES cell research with pre-existing coded or anonymous hES cell lines in general is permissible provided that notice of the research, documentation of the provenance of the cell lines, and evidence of compliance with any required Institutional Review Board, Institutional Animal Care and Use Committee, Institutional Biosafety Committee, or other mandated reviews is provided to the ESCRO committee or other body designated by the investigator's institution.

(b) Research that is permissible only after additional review and approval by an ESCRO committee or other equivalent body designated by the investigator's institution.
(i) The ESCRO committee should evaluate all requests for permission to attempt derivation of new hES cell lines from donated blastocysts, from *in vitro* fertilized oocytes, or by nuclear transfer. The scientific rationale for the need to generate new hES cell lines, by whatever means, should be clearly presented, and the basis for the numbers of blastocysts or oocytes needed should be justified. Such requests should be accompanied by evidence of Institutional Review Board approval of the procurement process.
(ii) All research involving the introduction of hES cells into nonhuman animals at any stage of embryonic, fetal, or postnatal development should be reviewed by the ESCRO committee. Particular attention should be paid to the probable pattern and effects of differentiation and integration of the human cells into the nonhuman animal tissues.
(iii) Research in which personally identifiable information about the donors of the blastocysts, gametes, or somatic cells from which the hES cells were derived is readily ascertainable by the investigator also requires ESCRO committee review and approval.

(c) Research that should not be permitted at this time:
(i) Research involving *in vitro* culture of any intact human embryo, regardless of derivation method, for longer than 14 days or until formation of the primitive streak begins, whichever occurs first.
(ii) Research in which hES cells are introduced into nonhuman primate blastocysts or in which any ES cells are introduced into human blastocysts.

In addition:
> (iii) No animal into which hES cells have been introduced at any stage of development should be allowed to breed.

Recommendation 4:
Through its Embryonic Stem Cell Research Oversight (ESCRO) committee, each research institution should establish and maintain a registry of investigators conducting hES cell research and record descriptive information about the types of research being performed and the hES cells in use.

Recommendation 5:
If a U.S.-based investigator collaborates with an investigator in another country, the Embryonic Stem Cell Research Oversight (ESCRO) committee may determine that the procedures prescribed by the foreign institution afford protections equivalent with these guidelines and may approve the substitution of some or all of the foreign procedures for its own.

Recommendation 6:
A national body should be established to assess periodically the adequacy of the guidelines proposed in this document and to provide a forum for a continuing discussion of issues involved in hES cell research.

Recommendation 7:
The hES cell research community should ensure that there is sufficient genetic diversity among cell lines to allow for potential translation into health-care services for all groups in our society.

RECOMMENDATIONS FROM CHAPTER 4

Recommendation 8:
Regardless of the source of funding and the applicability of federal regulations, an Institutional Review Board or its equivalent should review the procurement of gametes, blastocysts, or somatic cells for the purpose of generating new hES cell lines, including the procurement of blastocysts in excess of clinical need from *in vitro* fertilization clinics, blastocysts made through *in vitro* fertilization specifically for research purposes, and oocytes, sperm, and somatic cells donated for development of hES cell lines derived through nuclear transfer.

Recommendation 9:
Institutional Review Boards may not waive the requirement for obtaining informed consent from any person whose somatic cells, gametes, or blastocysts are used in hES research.

Recommendation 10:
Investigators, institutions, Institutional Review Boards, and privacy boards should ensure that authorizations are received from donors, as appropriate and required by federal human subjects protections and the Health Insurance Portability and Accountability Act for the confidential transmission of personal health information to repositories or to investigators who are using hES cell lines derived from donated materials.

Recommendation 11:
Investigators and institutions involved in hES cell research should conduct the research in accordance with all applicable laws and guidelines pertaining to recombinant DNA research and animal care. Institutions should consider adopting Good Laboratory Practice standards for some or all of their basic hES cell research.

Recommendation 12:
hES cell research leading to potential clinical application must be in compliance with all applicable Food and Drug Administration (FDA) regulations. If FDA requires that a link to the donor source be maintained, investigators and institutions must ensure that the confidentiality of the donor is protected, that the donor understands that a link will be maintained, and that, where applicable, federal human subjects protections and Health Insurance Portability and Accountability Act or other privacy protections are followed.

RECOMMENDATIONS FROM CHAPTER 5

Recommendation 13:
When donor gametes have been used in the *in vitro* fertilization process, resulting blastocysts may not be used for research without consent of all gamete donors.

Recommendation 14:
To facilitate autonomous choice, decisions related to the production of embryos for infertility treatment should be free of the influence of investigators who propose to derive or use hES cells in research. Whenever it is practicable, the attending physician responsible for the infertility treatment and the investigator deriving or proposing to use hES cells should not be the same person.

Recommendation 15:
No cash or in kind payments may be provided for donating blastocysts in excess of clinical need for research purposes.

Recommendation 16:
Women who undergo hormonal induction to generate oocytes specifically for research purposes (such as for nuclear transfer) should be reimbursed only for direct expenses incurred as a result of the procedure, as determined by an Institutional Review Board. No cash or in kind payments should be provided for donating oocytes for research purposes. Similarly, no payments should be made for donations of sperm for research purposes or of somatic cells for use in nuclear transfer.

Recommendation 17:
Consent for blastocyst donation should be obtained from each donor at the time of donation. Even people who have given prior indication of their intent to donate to research any blastocysts that remain after clinical care should nonetheless give informed consent at the time of donation. Donors should be informed that they retain the right to withdraw consent until the blastocysts are actually used in cell line derivation.

Recommendation 18:
In the context of donation of gametes or blastocysts for hES cell research, the informed consent process, should, at a minimum, provide the following information:

a. A statement that the blastocysts or gametes will be used to derive hES cells for research that may include research on human transplantation.
b. A statement that the donation is made without any restriction or direction regarding who may be the recipient of transplants of the cells derived, except in the case of autologous donation.
c. A statement as to whether the identities of the donors will be readily ascertainable to those who derive or work with the resulting hES cell lines.
d. If the identities of the donors are retained (even if coded), a statement as to whether donors wish to be contacted in the future to receive information obtained through studies of the cell lines.
e. An assurance that participants in research projects will follow applicable and appropriate best practices for donation, procurement, culture, and storage of cells and tissues to ensure, in particular, the traceability of stem cells. (Traceable information, however, must be secured to ensure confidentiality.)
f. A statement that derived hES cells and/or cell lines might be kept for many years.
g. A statement that the hES cells and/or cell lines might be used in research involving genetic manipulation of the cells or the mixing of human and nonhuman cells in animal models.

h. Disclosure of the possibility that the results of study of the hES cells may have commercial potential and a statement that the donor will not receive financial or any other benefits from any future commercial development;

i. A statement that the research is not intended to provide direct medical benefit to the donor(s) except in the case of autologous donation.

j. A statement that embryos will be destroyed in the process of deriving hES cells.

k. A statement that neither consenting nor refusing to donate embryos for research will affect the quality of any future care provided to potential donors.

l. A statement of the risks involved to the donor.

Recommendation 19:
Consenting or refusing to donate gametes or embryos for research should not affect or alter in any way the quality of care provided to prospective donors. That is, clinical staff must provide appropriate care to patients without prejudice regarding their decisions about disposition of their embryos.

Recommendation 20:
Clinical personnel who have a conscientious objection to hES cell research should not be required to participate in providing donor information or securing donor consent for research use of gametes or blastocysts. That privilege should not extend to the care of a donor or recipient.

Recommendation 21:
Researchers may not ask members of the infertility treatment team to generate more oocytes than necessary for the optimal chance of reproductive success. An infertility clinic or other third party responsible for obtaining consent or collecting materials should not be able to pay for or be paid for the material obtained (except for specifically defined cost-based reimbursements and payments for professional services).

Recommendation 22:
Institutions that are banking or plan to bank hES cell lines should establish uniform guidelines to ensure that donors of material give informed consent through a process approved by an Institutional Review Board, and that meticulous records are maintained about all aspects of cell culture. Uniform tracking systems and common guidelines for distribution of cells should be established.

Recommendation 23:
Any facility engaged in obtaining and storing hES cell lines should consider the following standards:

(a) Creation of a committee for policy and oversight purposes and creation of clear and standardized protocols for banking and withdrawals.
(b) Documentation requirements for investigators and sites that deposit cell lines, including
    (i)   A copy of the donor consent form.
    (ii)   Proof of Institutional Review Board approval of the procurement process.
    (iii) Available medical information on the donors, including results of infectious-disease screening.
    (iv) Available clinical, observational, or diagnostic information about the donor(s).
    (v)   Critical information about culture conditions (such as media, cell passage, and safety information).
    (vi) Available cell line characterization (such as karyotype and genetic markers).
A repository has the right of refusal if prior culture conditions or other items do not meet its standards.

(c) A secure system for protecting the privacy of donors when materials retain codes or identifiable information, including but not limited to
    (i)   A schema for maintaining confidentiality (such as a coding system).
    (ii)   A system for a secure audit trail from primary cell lines to those submitted to the repository.
    (iii) A policy governing whether and how to deliver clinically significant information back to donors.

(d) The following standard practices:
    (i)   Assignment of a unique identifier to each sample.
    (ii)   A process for characterizing cell lines.
    (iii) A process for expanding, maintaining, and storing cell lines.
    (iv) A system for quality assurance and control.
    (v)   A website that contains scientific descriptions and data related to the cell lines available.
    (vi) A procedure for reviewing applications for cell lines.
    (vii) A process for tracking disbursed cell lines and recording their status when shipped (such as number of passages).
    (viii) A system for auditing compliance.
    (ix) A schedule of charges.

(x)   A statement of intellectual property policies.
(xi) When appropriate, creation of a clear Material Transfer Agreement or user agreement.
(xii) A liability statement.
(xiii) A system for disposal of material.

(e) Clear criteria for distribution of cell lines, including but not limited to evidence of approval of the research by an Embryonic Stem Cell Research Oversight committee or equivalent body at the recipient institution.

Appendix B

Committee Biographies

Richard O. Hynes, PhD, (Co-Chair), (NAS, IOM) is the Daniel K. Ludwig Professor of Cancer Research at the MIT Center for Cancer Research and Department of Biology, and a Howard Hughes Medical Institute investigator. He was formerly head of the Biology Department and then director of the Center for Cancer Research. His research focuses on fibronectins and integrins and the molecular basis of cellular adhesion, both in normal development and in pathological situations, such as cancer, thrombosis, and inflammation. Dr. Hynes's current interests are cancer invasion and metastasis, angiogenesis, and animal models of human disease states. In 1997, he received the Gairdner International Foundation Award. In 2000, he served as president of the American Society for Cell Biology and testified before Congress about the need for federal support and oversight of embryonic stem cell research.

Jonathan D. Moreno, PhD, (Co-Chair), is the Emily Davie and Joseph S. Kornfeld Professor of Biomedical Ethics and director of the Center for Biomedical Ethics at the University of Virginia. He is a past president of the American Society for Bioethics and Humanities and is a member of the Council on Accreditation of the Association of Human Research Protection Programs. Dr. Moreno is also a member of the Board on Health Sciences Policy of the Institute of Medicine. Among Dr. Moreno's books are *In the Wake of Terror: Medicine and Morality in a Time of Crisis*, and *Undue Risk: Secret State Experiments on Humans*. Dr. Moreno also serves as a commentator and columnist for ABCNews.com and is a frequent guest on various news programs, including NBC Nightly News with Tom Brokaw. Dr. Moreno was a senior consultant for the National Bioethics Advisory Commission and a senior staff member of the Advisory Committee on Human Radiation Experiments during the Clinton administration.

Elizabeth Price Foley, JD, LLM, is a professor of law at Florida International University (FIU) College of Law. Before joining the FIU College of Law in 2002 as one of its founding faculty, she was a professor of law at Michigan State University (MSU) College of Law and an Adjunct Professor in the Center for Ethics and Humanities of the MSU College of Human Medicine. Dr. Foley's scholarship focuses on bioethics and the intersection of health care law and constitutional law, and her articles have been cited in more than 100 law journals. She is a frequent commentator on health law and bioethics issues for national and international media such as CNN, Fox News, the Washington Post, and the Wall Street Journal. Before teaching law, Dr. Foley served as a judicial clerk on the U.S. Court of Appeals for the Fifth Circuit. She also spent a number of years on Capitol Hill, serving as senior legislative aide to Representative Ron Wyden (D-OR), legislative aide for the District of Columbia office of the Health Insurance Plan of Greater New York, and legislative aide for Representative Michael Andrews (D-TX). Dr. Foley received her BA from Emory University, her JD from the University of Tennessee College of Law and her LLM from Harvard Law School.

Norman Fost, MD, MPH, is a professor of pediatrics and director of the Program in Bioethics, which he founded in 1973. He is chair of the Health Sciences Institutional Review Board, chair of the University of Wisconsin Hospital Ethics Committee, chair of the university's Bioethics Advisory Committee, and director of the Child Protection Team. He was a member of Hillary Clinton's Health Care Task Force and numerous other federal and state committees. He received his AB from Princeton, his MD from Yale, and his MPH from Harvard. He has been awarded the Nellie Westerman Prize in Research Ethics, and the William Bartholome Award for Excellence in Ethics from the American Academy of Pediatrics. His research interests include regulation of human subjects research, ethical and policy issues in access to human growth hormone, and the use of interactive computers in genetic counseling.

H. Robert Horvitz, PhD, (NAS, IOM) is the David H. Koch Professor of Biology in the Department of Biology at MIT and a Howard Hughes Medical Institute investigator. He is also a member of the McGovern Institute for Brain Research at MIT and a member of the MIT Center for Cancer Research. Dr. Horvitz's research interests include molecular and cellular biology, developmental and behavioral genetics, apoptosis, human neurological disease, neural development, morphogenesis, cell lineage, cell fate, micro-RNAs, signal transduction, transcriptional repression, and chromatin remodeling. Dr. Horvitz has served as a member of the Advisory Council of the National Human Genome Research Institute of the National Institutes of Health and was co-chair of the Working Group on Preclinical Models for

Cancer of the National Cancer Institute. He was President of the Genetics Society of America in 1995. Dr. Horvitz received the Charles A. Dana Award for Pioneering Achievements in Health (1995), the General Motors Cancer Research Foundation Alfred P. Sloan, Jr. Prize (1998), the Gairdner Foundation International Award (1999), and the Bristol-Myers Squibb Award for Distinguished Achievement in Neuroscience (2001). In 2002, he received the Nobel Prize in Physiology or Medicine for his studies of the genetic regulation of organ development and programmed cell death.

Marcia Imbrescia is the current owner of Peartree Design, a landscape firm, and was previously the media director for Drumbeater, a high technology advertising agency. She holds BA degrees in marketing and journalism, and a graduate certificate in landscape design. Ms. Imbrescia has a passion for health advocacy and helping people with illness and disability. She is a member of the Board of Trustees of the Arthritis Foundation (AF), for which she has participated as a volunteer at the chapter and national levels. She served as member (1996-1998, 2001) and chairperson (2002-2003) of AF's American Juvenile Arthritis Organization. In 1992, she received the Volunteer of the Year Award from the Massachusetts Chapter of AF. Her volunteer efforts include program development, conference planning, public speaking, fundraising, and advocacy.

Terry Magnuson, PhD, is Sarah Graham Kenan Professor and chair of the Department of Genetics at the University of North Carolina. He also directs the Carolina Center for Genome Sciences, and is the program director of cancer genetics at the Lineberger Comprehensive Cancer Center. Dr. Magnuson's research interests include mammalian genetics, genomics, and development. His laboratory has developed a high-throughput system to study the effects of mutations on mouse development with mouse embryonic stem cells. He is particularly interested in the role of murine polycomb-group genes on the processes of autosomal imprinting, X-inactivation, and anterior-posterior patterning of axial structures in mammals. He is a member of the Board of Directors of the Genetics Society of America and of the Society for Developmental Biology.

Cheryl Mwaria, PhD, is professor of anthropology and director of African studies at Hofstra University. Her fieldwork as a medical anthropologist in Kenya, Botswana, Namibia, the Caribbean, and the United States has focused on women's health, race relations, and differential access to health care. She has served on the Executive Boards of the American Ethnological Society, the Society for the Study of Anthropology of North America, and the Association of Feminist Anthropology. She is currently director of the Africa Network, a nonprofit consortium of liberal arts colleges committed to literacy about and concern for Africa in American higher education. Dr. Mwaria is a member of the Center for Urban Bioethics at the New York Academy of Medicine and has served as a consultant in community values in end-of-life care for North General Hospital in New York City and the New York Academy of Medicine Center for Urban Bioethics. Her most recent fieldwork (2002-2003) was conducted at a major cancer research center and focused on minority group access to cancer-related clinical trials. Her publications pertaining to biomedical ethics include "Biomedical Ethics, Gender and Ethnicity: Implications for Black Feminist Anthropology" in *Black Feminist Anthropology: Theory, Praxis, Politics and Poetics* (Irma McClaurin, ed., 2001).

Janet Rossant, PhD, is the co-head of the Fetal Health and Development Program at Mount Sinai Hospital, professor at the University of Toronto, and director of the Center for Modelling Human Disease. Dr. Rossant studies lineage determination in the developing embryo. She has received numerous prizes for her work in establishing the fates of early developing cells in the mouse embryo, including the McLaughlin Medal from the Royal Society of Canada, the Canadian Institute of Health Research (CIHR) Distinguished Scientist Award, and the Robert L. Noble Prize from the National Cancer Institute of Canada. She is a member of the Board of Directors of the International Society for Stem Cell Research and participated in the development of the CIHR guidelines for embryonic stem cell research, which do not permit the use of somatic cell nuclear transfer to create stem cells.

Janet D. Rowley, MD, (NAS, IOM) is the Blum-Riese Distinguished Service Professor in the Departments of Medicine, Molecular Genetics and Cell Biology, and Human Genetics at the University of Chicago. She has contributed significantly to advances in understanding of genetic changes in cancer. She focused on chromosomal abnormalities in human leukemia and lymphoma and in 1972, using new techniques of chromosome identification, discovered the first consistent chromosomal translocation in human cancer. She has identified more than a dozen recurring translocations. Her laboratory is analyzing the gene expression pattern of recurring translocations to identify unique markers of leukemias for diagnosis and potentially as therapeutic targets. With Felix Mitelman, she cofounded and is coeditor of *Genes, Chromosomes and Cancer*, the premier cancer cytogenetics journal. She is a member of the President's Council on Bioethics.

Liaison from the Board on Life Sciences

R. Alta Charo, JD, is the Elizabeth S. Wilson-Bascom Professor of Law and Bioethics at the University of Wisconsin Law and Medical Schools, and associate dean for research and faculty development at the University of Wisconsin Law School at Madison. She is the author of over 75 articles, book chapters, and government reports on such topics as voting rights, environmental law, reproductive rights, medical genetics law, reproductive technology policy, and science policy. She serves on the expert advisory boards of several organizations with an interest in stem cell research, including the Juvenile Diabetes Research Foundation, WiCell, and the Wisconsin Stem Cell Research Program. She is also a consultant to the California Institute for Regenerative Medicine. In 1994, Dr. Charo served on the National Institutes of Health Human Embryo Research Panel. From 1996 to 2001, she was a member of the National Bioethics Advisory Commission and participated in the writing of its reports on research ethics and cloning. Since 2001, she has been a member of the National Academies Board on Life Sciences.

Appendix C

Workshop Agenda and Speaker Biographies

Board on Life Sciences
The National Academies
and
Board on Health Sciences Policy
Institute of Medicine

Guidelines for Human Embryonic Stem Cell Research

Public Workshop

Agenda, Tuesday, October 12, 2004
Main Auditorium
National Academy of Sciences
2101 Constitution Ave., NW   Washington, D.C.

8:30 a.m.   **Welcome:** Bruce Alberts, President, National Academy of Sciences
Harvey Fineberg, President, Institute of Medicine

8:45 a.m.   **Introduction and Mandate of the Committee on Guidelines for Human Embryonic Stem Cell Research:**

Richard Hynes, Massachusetts Institute of Technology and Co-Chair, Committee on Guidelines for Human Embryonic Stem Cell Research

9:00 a.m.   **Overview of the Human Embryonic Stem Cell Science and Policy Issues**

Moderator: Richard Hynes

- Stem Cell Science—Where Have We Come From, Where Are We Going?
  Martin Raff, University College London

- Overview of Policies and Rules—An International Perspective
  LeRoy Walters, Georgetown University

- Discussant: Anne McLaren, Centre for Medical Genetics and Policy, University of Cambridge

9:50 a.m.   **Q & A**

10:15 a.m.   Break

10:30 a.m.   **Derivation and Use of Human Embryonic Stem Cells—General Issues**
Moderator: Janet Rossant, Mount Sinai Hospital, Toronto

Panel: George Daley, Harvard Medical School
            Fred (Rusty) Gage, the Salk Institute

Discussants: James Battey, National Institutes of Health
               Leonard Zon, Harvard Medical School

11:30 p.m. **Q & A**

12:00 p.m. Lunch

1:00 p.m.   **Stem Cells and Somatic Cell Nuclear Transfer**

Moderator: H. Robert Horvitz, MIT and Howard Hughes Medical Institute

Panel: Rudolf Jaenisch, Whitehead Institute
        Davor Solter, Max Planck Institute of Immunobiology

Discussant: Kevin Eggan, Harvard University

1:50 p.m.   Q&A

2:20 p.m.   Break

2:35 p.m.   **Interspecies Mixing and Chimeras**

                Moderator: Terry Magnusson, University of North Carolina

                Panel: Irving Weissman, Stanford University School of Medicine
                       David Garbers, University of Texas Southwestern Medical
                       Center at Dallas

                Discussant: Brigid Hogan, Duke University

3:25 p.m.   Q&A

3:55 p.m.   **Current Legal and Regulatory Requirements That May Affect
Human Embryonic Stem Cell Research**

                Panel: Alta Charo, University of Wisconsin School of Law
                    Michael Malinowski, Louisiana State University School of
                    Law

4:35 p.m.   Q&A

5:00 p.m.   Public Comment

5:30 p.m.   **Adjourn**

Agenda, Wednesday, October 13, 2004
Lecture Room
National Academy of Sciences
2101 Constitution Ave., NW Washington, D.C.

8:30 a.m.   **Opening Remarks:** Jonathan Moreno, University of Virginia, and
Co-Chair, Committee on Guidelines for Human Embryonic Stem
Cell Research

8:45 a.m.   **Informed Consent and Procurement**

Moderator: Jonathan Moreno

Presentation: Ruth Faden, Phoebe R. Berman Bioethics Institute, Johns Hopkins University

Discussants: Alison Murdoch, Department of Reproductive Medicine, International Centre for Life
Catherine Racowsky, Brigham and Women's Hospital, Division of Reproductive Medicine

9:25 a.m.   Q&A

9:40 a.m.   **Derivation of Stem Cell Lines—Ethics and Policy Concerns**

Moderator: Janet Rowley, University of Chicago

• Panel on SCNT for human embryonic stem cell research
Dan Brock, Harvard Medical School
Leon Kass, President's Council on Bioethics

• Panel on species mixing/chimeras for human embryonic stem cell research
Henry Greely, Stanford Law School
Cynthia Cohen, Georgetown University
William Hurlbut, Stanford University (20 minutes)

11:20 a.m.   Q&A

11:45 a.m.   **Patenting, Licensing, and Material Transfer Agreements in Relation to Human Embryonic Stem Cell Research**

Moderator: Elizabeth Price Foley, Florida International University College of Law

Presentation: Carl Gulbrandsen, Wisconsin Alumni Research Foundation

12:15 p.m.   Q&A

12:30 p.m.   Lunch

1:05 p.m.   **Mechanisms for Oversight of Human Embryonic Stem Cell Research**

              Moderator: Norman Fost, University of Wisconsin

              Panel: Laurie Zoloth, Center for Genetic Medicine, Northwestern University
              Franco Furger, Executive Director, Human Biotechnology Governance Forum, Johns Hopkins University

1:40 p.m.   Q&A

1:55 p.m.   **Industry Perspective: What Is Industry's Role in Monitoring the Ethics of Human Embryonic Stem Cell Research?**

              Moderator: Marcia Imbrescia, Arthritis Foundation Board of Trustees

              Presentation: Michael Werner, Chief of Policy, Biotechnology Industry Organization

2:15 p.m.   Q&A

2:30 p.m.   **Serving the Public Interest: Conducting Human Embryonic Stem Cell Research in a Democratic Society**

              Moderator: Cheryl Mwaria, Hofstra University

              • Panel: Dan Hausman, University of Wisconsin
              Robert Goldstein, Juvenile Diabetes Research Foundation
              Bruce Jennings, The Hastings Institute

3:30 p.m.   Q&A

3:45 p.m.   Public Comment

4:15 p.m.   **Summary and Concluding Remarks:**
              Jonathan Moreno and Richard Hynes

4:30 p.m.   Adjourn

SPEAKER BIOGRAPHIES

James F. Battey, Jr., MD, PhD, received his BS in physics from the California Institute of Technology in 1974 and his MD and PhD in biophysics from Stanford University School of Medicine in 1980. After receiving training in pediatrics, Dr. Battey pursued a postdoctoral fellowship in genetics at Harvard Medical School under the mentorship of Philip Leder. Since completing his postdoctoral fellowship in 1983, he has held a variety of positions at the National Institutes of Health, serving in the National Cancer Institute, the National Institute of Neurological Disorders and Stroke, and the National Institute on Deafness and Other Communication Disorders, of which he is currently the director. Until recently he also served as the chair of the NIH Stem Cell Task Force.

Dan W. Brock, PhD, is a former senior scientist and member of the Department of Clinical Bioethics at the National Institutes of Health and former professor of philosophy and biomedical ethics at Brown University, where he was also the Charles C. Tillinghast, Jr. University Professor, professor of philosophy and biomedical ethics, and director of the Center for Biomedical Ethics through June 2002. He is professor of medical ethics in the Department of Social Science at Harvard Medical School. Dr. Brock works on such subjects as genes and justice, health care resource prioritization and rationing, and end of life care and euthanasia. He has published numerous papers in bioethics and in moral and political philosophy. His most recent works include "Priority to the Worst Off in Health Care Resource Prioritization" and "Broadening the Bioethics Agenda." He is also the author of *Deciding For Others: The Ethics of Surrogate Decision Making* (with Allen E. Buchanan, 1989); *Life and Death: Philosophical Essays in Biomedical Ethics* (1993); and *From Chance to Choice: Genetics and Justice* (with Allen Buchanan, Norman Daniels, and Daniel Wikler, 2000).

R. Alta Charo, JD, is the Elizabeth S. Wilson-Bascom Professor of Law and Bioethics at the University of Wisconsin Law and Medical Schools, and Associate Dean for Research and Faculty Development at the University of Wisconsin Law School at Madison. Professor Charo is the author of over 75 articles, book chapters, and government reports on topics including voting rights, environmental law, reproductive rights, medical genetics law, reproductive technology policy, and science policy. She serves on the expert advisory boards of several organizations with an interest in stem cell research, including the Juvenile Diabetes Research Foundation, WiCell, and the Wisconsin Stem Cell Research Program. She is also a consultant to the California Institute for Regenerative Medicine. In 1994, Professor Charo served on the NIH Human Embryo Research Panel, and from 1996-2001 she was a member of the presidential National Bioethics Advisory Commission, where she participated in writing its reports on research ethics and cloning. Since 2001 she has been a member of the National Academies' Board on Life Sciences.

Cynthia Cohen, PhD, JD, is a faculty affiliate of the Kennedy Institute of Ethics at Georgetown University in Washington, D.C., and a fellow at the Hastings Center in Garrison, New York. She is the former executive director of the National Advisory Board on Ethics in Reproduction in Washington, DC, associate for ethical studies at the Hastings Center, associate to the legal counsel of the University of Michigan Hospitals, and chair of the Philosophy Department at the University of Denver. She is a member of the Canadian Stem Cell Oversight Committee and has served as a consultant to such groups as the National Institutes of Health, the American Association for the Advancement of Science, and the Stem Cell Network. Dr. Cohen has written or edited eight books and some 150 articles on ethical issues, including stem cell research, genetic testing, reproductive and therapeutic cloning, the new reproductive technologies, organ transplantation, mandatory drug testing, and religion and public policy.

George Q. Daley, MD, PhD, is an associate professor of biological chemistry and molecular pharmacology at Harvard Medical School. He received a bachelor's degree (1982) from Harvard University, his PhD (1989) in biology from the Massachusetts Institute of Technology (MIT), and his MD (1991) from Harvard Medical School through the Harvard-MIT Division of Health Sciences and Technology. Dr. Daley's laboratory studies stem cell development and differentiation, emphasizing derivation of functional hematopoietic and germ cell elements from embryonic stem cells and the genetic mechanisms that predispose to malignancy. Dr. Daley is Board Certified in Internal Medicine and Hematology, and is a staff physician in Hematology/Oncology at the Children's Hospital, the Dana Farber Cancer Institute, and the Brigham and Women's Hospital in Boston. He has been elected to the American Society for Clinical Investigation and has received research awards from Harvard Medical School, the National Institutes of Health, the New England Cancer Society, the Burroughs Wellcome Fund, the Edward Mallinckrodt, Jr. Foundation, and the Leukemia and Lymphoma Society of America. Dr. Daley was recently named a recipient of the NIH Director's Pioneer Award, an unrestricted grant to pursue highly innovative avenues of research.

Kevin Eggan, PhD, is a junior fellow in the Harvard Society of Fellows at Harvard University, having recently completed postdoctoral studies in the laboratory of Rudy Jaenisch at the Whitehead Institute for Biomedical Research. At Harvard, Dr. Eggan is establishing an independent research group to study the molecular and genetic control of mouse preimplantation development, investigate epigenetic reprogramming after somatic cell nuclear transfer, and derive disease-specific human embryonic stem cell lines from diabetic and Parkinson's disease patients by nuclear transfer. Dr. Eggan has been invited to present his work at numerous symposia and workshops. He received a BS degree from the University of Illinois and a PhD from the Massachusetts Institute of Technology.

Ruth Faden, MPH, PhD, (IOM) is the Philip Franklin Wagley Professor of Biomedical Ethics and executive director of the Phoebe R. Berman Bioethics Institute at Johns Hopkins University. She is also a senior research scholar at the Kennedy Institute of Ethics, Georgetown University. Dr. Faden is the author and editor of numerous books and articles on biomedical ethics and health policy, including *A History and Theory of Informed Consent* (with Tom L. Beauchamp), *AIDS, Women and the Next Generation* (Ruth Faden, Gail Geller, and Madison Powers, eds.), and *HIV, AIDS and Childbearing: Public Policy, Private Lives* (Ruth Faden and Nancy Kass, eds.). She is a fellow of the Hastings Center and the American Psychological Association. She has served on several national advisory committees and commissions including the President's Advisory Committee on Human Radiation Experiments, which she chaired. Dr. Faden holds a BA from the University of Pennsylvania, an MA in general studies in humanities from the University of Chicago, and an MPH and PhD (Program in Attitudes and Behavior) from the University of California, Berkeley.

Franco Furger, PhD, is the executive director of the Human Biotechnology Governance Forum at the Foreign Policy Institute of the Paul H. Nitze School of Advanced International Studies at Johns Hopkins University. The 2-year project is exploring options for controlling research in and applications of "reprogenetics," research activities that focus on the beginning of life and procedures aimed at preventing the inheritance of genetic diseases. Such research activities include research cloning, stem cell research, and preimplantation genetic diagnosis. Before joining Johns Hopkins, he was a member of the faculty of George Mason University's School of Public Policy. Dr. Furger received an MS in electrical engineering in 1982 and a PhD in environmental sciences in 1992 from the Federal Institute of Technology in Zurich.

Fred H. Gage, PhD, (NAS) is a professor in the Laboratory of Genetics at the Salk Institute in La Jolla, California, and a professor of neuroscience at the University of California, San Diego. Dr. Gage received his undergraduate degree from the University of Florida and a PhD from Johns Hopkins University and is known for his discovery of structural and functional plasticity in the adult mammalian brain. His research focuses on the development of strategies to induce recovery of function after central nervous system damage and on the unexpected plasticity and adaptability that remain throughout the life of all mammals. His work may lead to methods of replacing brain tissue lost to stroke or Alzheimer's disease and repairing spinal cords damaged by trauma. Dr. Gage's laboratory showed that, contrary to years of dogma, human beings are capable of growing new nerve cells throughout life. Dr. Gage is a past president of the Society for Neuroscience. Among the awards he has received are the Charles A. Dana Award for Pioneering Achievements in Health and Education (1993), the Christopher Reeve Research Medal (1997), and the Max Planck Research Prize (1999).

David Garbers, PhD, is professor of pharmacology at the University of Texas Southwestern Medical Center in Dallas, Texas, and director of the Cecil H. and Ida Green Center for Reproductive Biology Sciences. He is also a Howard Hughes Medical Institute investigator. His laboratory explores how cells communicate with each other, particularly the mechanisms by which mammalian sperm detect signals from the egg. His research includes the development of technology to produce germ cells in vitro and to understand the mechanisms by which the mammalian egg is capable of reprogramming a somatic cell nucleus. He is a member of the American Academy of Arts and Sciences and has served on the editorial boards of various scientific journals, including the *Journal of Biological Chemistry, Biology of Reproduction,* and *Biochemical Journal and Endocrine Reviews.* Dr. Garbers received his bachelor's, master's, and PhD degrees in science from the University of Wisconsin. In 2001, he received the Endocrine Society's Edwin B. Astwood award.

Robert A Goldstein, MD, PhD, is the chief scientific officer of the Juvenile Diabetes Research Foundation International, where he is responsible for developing and guiding the research agenda. Before joining the foundation in 1997, he was director of the Division of Allergy, Immunology and Transplantation at the National Institute of Allergy and Infectious Diseases. He received his undergraduate degree from Brandeis University, his MD from Jefferson Medical College, his PhD in microbiology and immunology from George Washington University, and an MBA from the Stern School of Business, New York University. He recently testified before Congress on stem cell research.

Henry T. Greely, JD, is the Deane F. and Kate Edelman Johnson Professor of Law and a professor, by courtesy, of genetics at Stanford University. He specializes in legal and social issues arising from advances in the biological sciences and in health law and policy. He has written on genetic testing, human cloning, the ethics of human genetics research, legal issues in neuroscience, and policy issues in the health care financing system. He directs the Stanford Center for Law and the Biosciences, chairs the steering committee of the Stanford University Center for Biomedical Ethics, and co-directs the Stanford Program on Genomics, Ethics, and Society. Dr. Greely graduated from Stanford in 1974 and from Yale Law School in 1977. He joined the Stanford faculty in 1985.

Carl Gulbrandsen, PhD, JD, is the managing director of the Wisconsin Alumni Research Foundation (WARF) at the University of Wisconsin, Madison. He received his undergraduate degree from St. Olaf College in Northfield, Minnesota, a PhD in physiology from the University of Wisconsin, Madison, and a JD degree from the University of Wisconsin Law School. In 1992, after 9 years of private practice law focusing on intellectual property rights, Dr. Gulbrandsen joined Madison, WI companies Lunar Corporation and Bone Care International, Inc. as general counsel. He joined WARF in October 1997 as director of patents and licensing and in 2000 he became the managing director. He is a member of the Association of University Technology Managers, the Licensing Executive Society, the American Intellectual Property Law Association, the Wisconsin State Bar, and the American Bar Association. He is also a director of the WiCell Research Institute, the Cornell Research Foundation, and the Wisconsin Biotechnology Association.

Dan Hausman, PhD, is Herbert A. Simon Professor in the Department of Philosophy of the University of Wisconsin. After graduating from Harvard in 1969, where he studied biochemistry and then English history and literature, he taught public school in New York City and received a Master of Arts in Teaching from New York University. He then received a BA in philosophy from Cambridge University and a PhD from Columbia University in 1978. His dissertation (later published as *Capital, Profits and Prices*) addressed questions in the philosophy of science raised by economics, and a large portion of his research has focused on economic methodology. Partly as a result of editing the journal *Economics and Philosophy* (in 1984-1994, jointly with Michael McPherson), he has worked on issues in ethics and economics and foundational questions concerning the nature of rationality. His interest in economic methodology has led to a long and continuing research interest concerning the nature of causation.

Brigid Hogan, PhD, (IOM) is the George Barth Geller Professor and chair of the Department of Cell Biology, Duke University Medical Center. Before joining Duke, Dr. Hogan was a Howard Hughes Medical Institute investigator and Hortense B. Ingram Professor in the Department of Cell Biology at Vanderbilt University Medical Center. Dr. Hogan earned her PhD in biochemistry at the University of Cambridge. She was then a postdoctoral fellow in the Department of Biology at MIT. Before moving to the United States in 1988, Dr. Hogan was head of the Molecular Embryology Laboratory at the National Institute for Medical Research in London. Her research focuses on the genetic control of embryonic development and morphogenesis, using the mouse as a model system. Her laboratory developed methods for deriving mouse pluripotent embryonic germ cell lines. She was co-chair for science of the 1994 National Institutes of Health Human Embryo Research Panel and a member of the National Academies Panel on Scientific and Medical Aspects of Human Cloning. In the past few years, Dr. Hogan has been elected to the Royal Society of London, the American Academy of Arts and Sciences, and the Institute of Medicine.

William Hurlbut, MD, is a physician and consulting professor in the Program on Human Biology at Stanford University, where he has cotaught integrative courses with Luca Cavelli-Sforza on human genetic diversity and with Nobelist Baruch Blumberg on epidemics, evolution, and ethics. Dr. Hurlbut's main interests involve ethical issues associated with advancing biotechnology and neuroscience and the integration of philosophy of biology with Christian theology. His recent work has focused on the evolutionary origins of religious, spiritual, and moral awareness. In 2002, Dr. Hurlbut was appointed to the President's Council on Bioethics. He is a member of the Chemical and Biological Warfare working group of Stanford's Center for Security and International Cooperation. Dr. Hurlbut received his MD from Stanford and later conducted theological studies at Stanford and the Institute Catholique, Paris. His recent writings include *From Biology to Biography: The Science of the Human Person,* a chapter in Blankenhorn, D., Benson, I.T. and O'Hara, M. (eds.) *Who are We?: Essays on the Nature of the Human Person* (in press, 2004).

Rudolf Jaenisch, MD, (NAS) is a founding member of the Whitehead Institute and professor of biology at the Massachusetts Institute of Technology. Born in Germany, he received his MD from the University of Munich in 1967 and was a postdoctoral fellow first at the Max Planck Institute for Biochemistry, Munich, and then at Princeton University. After a period as a visiting fellow at the Institute for Cancer Research in Philadelphia, Dr. Jaenisch joined the Salk Institute in La Jolla, California, where he remained from 1972 to 1977, rising from assistant to associate research professor. In 1977 he returned to Germany, where until 1984 (when he joined the Whitehead Institute) he was head of the Department of Tumor Virology at the Heinrich Pette Institute for Experimental Virology and Immunology at the University of Hamburg. Dr. Jaenisch is a pioneer in transgenic science (making mouse models of human disease) whose methods have been used to explore the role of DNA modification, genomic imprinting, and X chromosome inactivation, which are important topics in the study of cancer, developmental processes, and neurological and connective tissue disorders. Dr. Jaenisch has made major contributions to the study of genomic reprogramming that occurs during nuclear cloning. In addition to receiving many awards for his work, he was elected to the U.S. National Academy of Sciences in 2003.

Bruce Jennings, MA, is senior research scholar at the Hastings Center. From 1991 through 1999, he served as the Center's executive vice president. He has directed several research projects on the care of the dying, health policy, chronic illness and long-term care, and ethical issues in human genetics. He served as associate director of a project that produced the widely cited and influential *Guidelines on the Termination of Life-Sustaining Treatment and the Care of the Dying.* With Mildred Z. Solomon of the Education Development Center in Newton, Massachusetts, he is cofounder of the Decisions Near the End of Life Program, a hospital-based educational program for physicians and other health professionals that has been used in over 200 hospitals in 30 states. Mr. Jennings has served as a consultant to several government and private organizations, including the American Hospital Association, the Education Development Center, the Robert Wood Johnson Foundation, the New York Academy of Medicine, the Prudential Foundation, and Eli Lilly and Company. He serves on the boards of directors of such organizations as the National Hospice and Palliative Care Organization, American Health Decisions, the American Association of Bioethics (1994-1997), and the Association of Politics and the Life Sciences. Mr. Jennings also serves on bioethics advisory committees for the Alzheimer's Association, the Episcopal Church of the United States, and the National Hospice and Palliative Care Organization. In addition to his work with the Hastings Center, Mr. Jennings teaches at the Yale University School of Medicine in the Department of Epidemiology and Public Health.

Leon Kass, MD, PhD, is Hertog Fellow in Social Thought at the American Enterprise Institute and is the Addie Clark Harding Professor at the College and the Committee on Social Thought at the University of Chicago (on leave of absence). He earned his BS and MD degrees at the University of Chicago (1958 and1962) and his PhD in biochemistry at Harvard (1967). After conducting molecular biology research at the National Institutes of Health while serving in the U.S. Public Health Service, Dr. Kass turned to the ethical and philosophical issues raised by biomedical advances and, more recently, to broader moral and cultural issues. From 1970 to 1972, Dr. Kass served as executive secretary of the Committee on the Life Sciences and Social Policy of the National Research Council, whose report *Assessing Biomedical Technologies* provided one of the first overviews of the emerging moral and social questions posed by biomedical advance. He taught at St. John's College, Annapolis, MD, and served as Joseph P. Kennedy Sr. Research Professor in Bioethics at the Kennedy Institute of Ethics at Georgetown University before returning in 1976 to the University of Chicago. His widely reprinted essays on biomedical ethics have dealt with issues raised by *in vitro* fertilization, cloning, genetic screening and genetic technology, organ transplantation, aging research, euthanasia and assisted suicide, and the moral nature of the medical profession. In 2001, Dr. Kass was appointed by President Bush to chair the President's Council on Bioethics.

Michael Malinowski, JD, is the Ernest and Iris Eldred Professor of Law, and associate director of the Program in Law, Science, and Public Health at the Paul M. Hebert Law Center at Louisiana State University. He is cofounder of the Program in Law, Medicine, and BioScience and chair of the Health and Human Services Committee of the American Bar Association (ABA). He is a member of the ABA President's Special Committee on Bioethics, Phi Beta Kappa, and Oxford University's 21st Century Trust. In 1999-2000, Dr. Malinowski was a SmithKline Beecham Distinguished Fellow in Law and Genetics at the Center for the Study of Law, Science and Technology and a visiting professor of law at the Arizona State University College of Law. Previously, he was counsel to the law firm of Foley, Hoag & Eliot LLP in Boston, where his practice focused on biotechnology and health care.

He received a BA from Tufts University and a JD from Yale Law School. After law school, he clerked for a year for the Honorable Emilio M. Garza and a year for the Honorable Carolyn Dineen King, both federal appellate judges on the U.S. Court of Appeals for the Fifth Circuit. While clerking for Judge King, he was an adjunct professor of law in the Health Law Institute at the University of Houston Law Center. Dr. Malinowski has served as a member of the Special Committee on Genetic Information Policy of the Commonwealth of Massachusetts; the Grant Advisory Committee for the Ethical, Legal, and Social Issues Joint Working Group for the Human Genome Project; and the Biotechnology Industry Organization's Bioethics Committee and Working Group on Biomedical Information. He has published extensively on the commercialization of biotechnology and related health care issues, including a recent piece, "Choosing the Genetic Makeup of Children: Our Eugenics Past, Present, and Future?" (36 Connecticut L. Rev. 125-224, 2003), and lectured on these topics throughout the United States, Europe, and Canada.

Anne McLaren, DBE, PhD, FRS, is a principal research associate at the Wellcome Trust/Cancer Research UK Gurdon Institute at the University of Cambridge and a member of the European Molecular Biology Organization (EMBO). Before joining the Institute in 1992, she spent 19 years as director of the Medical Research Council's Mammalian Development Unit in London. For the previous 15 years, she worked for the Agriculture Research Council in C. H. Waddington's Institute of Animal Genetics in Edinburgh. Dr. McLaren's research interests include developmental biology, reproductive biology, and genetics, including molecular genetics. Her primary model is the laboratory mouse and she is working on the development of mouse primordial germ cells and the pluripotent stem cells derived from them. Dr. McLaren was a member of the UK government's Warnock Committee on Human Fertilisation and Embryology and until the end of 2001 was a member of the UK Human Fertilisation and Embryology Authority, which regulates *in vitro* fertilization and human embryo research in the UK. She chaired the Scientific and Technical Advisory Group of the World Health Organization's Human Reproduction Programme and was a member of the Nuffield Foundation's Bioethics Council. She is a member of the European Group on Ethics, which advises the European Commission on social and ethical implications of new technologies. Dr. McLaren, who completed her undergraduate and graduate work at Oxford University, was elected a fellow of the Royal Society in 1975 and she has served as the Society's Foreign Secretary and Vice-President. She is a founding member of Academia Europaea and of the recently established Academy of Medical Sciences. In 2002, she was awarded (jointly with A. K. Tarkowski) the Japan Prize for Developmental Biology.

Alison Murdoch, MD, FRCOG, is a consultant gynecologist and professor of reproductive medicine and the head of the Newcastle Fertility Centre for Life of the International Centre for Life at Newcastle University. Dr. Murdoch received her

BSc in medical science from Edinburgh University in 1972, followed by an MBChB (Bachelor of Medicine, Bachelor of Surgery) in 1975, an MD degree in 1987, and an FRCOG (Fellow of the Royal College of Obstetricians and Gynecologists) in 2001. Dr. Murdoch has been a speaker at such prestigious events as the International Conference on IVF in Chennai in 2001, the Stem Cell Research BFS/RCOG Ethics Meeting in 2002, and the Indian Medical Association Conference in Mangalore in September 2002. She was a guest lecturer at the medical staff rounds at Hammersmith Hospital in February 2003, a speaker at the British Council Symposium at the International Centre for Life in March 2003, the Updates in Infertility Conference in Florida in 2004, and she was the Keynote speaker at the British Congress of Obstetrics and Gynecology in Glasgow in 2004. In addition to her work at the Fertility Centre for Life, Dr. Murdoch is the chair of the British Fertility Society, an inspector for the Human Fertilisation and Embryology Authority, and a member of a panel that gave evidence to the House of Lords Select Committee on Stem Cell Research.

Catherine Racowsky, PhD, is the director of Assisted Reproductive Technologies (ART) Laboratory in the Department of Obstetrics, Gynecology and Reproductive Biology at the Center for Reproductive Medicine, Brigham and Women's Hospital. She is also an associate professor at Harvard University. Dr. Racowsky received her BA from the University of Oxford and her PhD from the University of Cambridge. Before joining Harvard and Brigham and Women's, her academic appointments included the University of Arizona Department of Animal Sciences, Department of Physiology, and Center of Toxicology. She served as the director of research in the Department of Obstetrics, Gynecology and Reproductive Biology in the College of Medicine at the University of Arizona and also director of the ART Laboratory. She is a full member of the Canadian Andrology and Fertility Society. From 1997 through 2001, she was a Member of the Reproductive Toxicology Editorial Board. She received the 2000 Partners Healthcare Excellence Award in Leadership and Innovation. Her research focuses on the effects of caffeine and smoking on human fertility. She has recently spoken at such diverse places as the Jones Institute in Norfolk, Virginia, on the topic "Embryo Selection: Can It Be Improved?" and the Taiwanese Society for Reproductive Medicine in Taipei, Taiwan, on the topics "Quality Management of the IVF Laboratory" and "Embryo Selection and Its Impact on How Many Embryos to Transfer."

Martin Raff, MD, (NAS) is a professor in the Department of Biology of the Medical Research Council MRC Laboratory for Molecular and Cell Biology at University College London. He received his BSc and MD from McGill University. He then pursued residencies in medicine at the Royal Victoria Hospital in Montreal and in neurology at Massachusetts General Hospital in Boston. Dr. Raff completed his postdoctoral training in immunology at the National Institute for Medical Research in London, after which he moved to University College London and has been a professor of biology since 1979. He is a Fellow of the Royal Society and of Academia Europaea, a foreign member of the American Academy of Arts and Sciences, and past president of the British Society of Cell Biology. His research interests span immunology, cell biology, and developmental neurobiology. Using the retina and optic nerve as model systems, he discovered that animal cells live, grow, differentiate, or proliferate depending on a combination of cell-cell interactions and cell-intrinsic programs. Dr. Raff is a foreign associate of the U.S. National Academy of Sciences.

Davor Solter, MD, PhD, is the director and a member of the Max Planck Institute of Immunobiology. He is also a senior staff scientist at the Jackson Laboratory in Bar Harbor, Maine, and an adjunct professor at the Wistar Institute in Philadelphia. Dr. Solter received his MSc, MD, and PhD from the University of Zagreb. He serves as a member of numerous editorial and advisory boards and is the European editor of *Genes and Development*. He is a member of the American Academy of Arts and Sciences, the European Molecular Biology Organization, and Academia Europea. In 1998, he received the March of Dimes Prize in Developmental Biology for pioneering the concept of imprinting, and in 1999, he was distinguished as a J. W. Jenkinson Memorial Lecturer at Oxford University. Dr. Solter has contributed to many fields of mammalian developmental biology, including the differentiation of germ layers, the role of cell surface molecules in regulating early development, the biology and genetics of teratocarcinoma, the biology of embryonic stem cells, and imprinting and cloning. His current research focuses on genetic and molecular control of genome reprogramming and of activation of the embryonic genome.

LeRoy Walters, PhD, is the Joseph P. Kennedy, Sr. Professor of Christian Ethics at the Kennedy Institute of Ethics, Georgetown University, and a professor of philosophy at Georgetown. He is coauthor with Julie Gage Palmer of *The Ethics of Human Gene Therapy* (1997), coeditor with Tom L. Beauchamp of an anthology titled *Contemporary Issues in Bioethics* (6th ed., 2003) and coeditor with Tamar Joy Kahn and Doris M. Goldstein of the annual *Bibliography of Bioethics* (1975-present). From 1965 through 1967, he studied at the University of Heidelberg and the Free University of Berlin. In 1971, he received his PhD from Yale University. Since 1999, Dr. Walters has had an active interest in human embryonic stem cell research. He served as a consultant to the National Bioethics Advisory Committee in 1999 and discussed ethical issues in human embryonic stem cell research at a National Academy of Sciences workshop in June 2001. In August 2001, he was consulted by President Bush on public policies for stem cell research. His most recent article, published in the March 2004 issue of the *Kennedy Institute of Ethics Journal*, was "Human Embryonic Stem Cell Research: An Intercultural Perspective."

Irving L. Weissman, MD, PhD, (NAS, IOM) is the Karel and Avice Bekhuis Professor of Cancer Biology and professor of pathology and developmental biology at Stanford University. He is cofounder and director of StemCells, Inc., a company focused on adult stem cell biology. Dr. Weissman's research interests encompass developmental biology, self-renewal, homing, and functions of the cells that make up the blood-forming and immune systems. His main focus for the last several years has been the purification, biology, transplantation, and evolution of stem cells. The isolation of mouse hematopoietic stem cells (HSC) in his laboratory was followed by the isolation of human HSCs by Dr. Weissman and his colleagues at SyStemix, Inc., of which he was a founder. Purified human HSCs have been successfully used to provide cancer-free autologous stem cell transplants for patients receiving otherwise lethal chemotherapy and radiotherapy for cancer. His laboratory has gone on to identify the stages of development between stem cells and mature blood cells. Dr. Weissman is the recipient of several awards, including the Leukemia Society of America de Villier's International Achievement Award, the E. Donnall Thomas Prize from the American Society of Hematology, and the Montana Conservationist of the Year Award.

Michael J. Werner is chief of policy for the Biotechnology Industry Organization (BIO), overseeing all policy development, legislative, regulatory, bioethics, and legal department activities. Before becoming chief of policy, Mr. Werner was BIO's vice president of bioethics. In that capacity, he led BIO's efforts to develop policies, programs, and activities that promote responsible and ethical uses of biotechnology. His work has explored a variety of bioethics issues, including, confidentiality of medical information, use of genetic information, gene therapy, cloning, stem cell research, xenotransplantation, protection of human subjects in research, and global health. Mr. Werner has over 17 years of experience in health law and policy in Washington, DC. Before joining BIO, he spent 6 years as counsel for legislation and policy for the American College of Physicians-American Society of Internal Medicine, performing legal analysis, policy development, and congressional and regulatory advocacy on a variety of issues, including end of life care, Medicare reform, liability reform, and integration and delivery system re-structuring. Mr. Werner also served as a senior health adviser to US Senate Majority Leader George Mitchell and as senior adviser to Maryland Governor William Donald Schaefer.

Laurie Zoloth, PhD, is professor of medical ethics and humanities and of religion at the Feinberg School of Medicine of Northwestern University. Her research projects include work on emerging issues in medical and research genetics, ethical issues in stem cell research, and distributive justice in health care. Dr. Zoloth chairs the Howard Hughes Medical Institute's Bioethics Advisory Board and served as president of the American Society for Bioethics and Humanities in 2001. She is a member of numerous advisory boards including, the National Aeronautics and Space Administration National Advisory Council; the Executive Committee of the

International Society for Stem Cell Research; the American Association of the Advancement of Science's (AAAS) Dialogue on Science, Ethics and Religion; the Geron Ethics Advisory Board; the Data Safety Monitoring Board for the National Institutes of Health International AIDS Clinical Trials Group; the AAAS Working Group on Human Germ-Line Interventions and on Stem Cell Research; and the Ethics Section of the American Academy of Religion. In 1999, she was invited to give testimony to the National Bioethics Advisory Board on Jewish philosophy and stem cell research. In 2001, she was named principal investigator for the International Project on Judaism and Genetics, cosponsored by the AAAS and supported by the Haas Foundation and the Greenwall Foundation. Dr. Zoloth received a BA in Women's Studies and History from the University of California at Berkeley, a BSN from the State University of New York, an MA in English from San Francisco State University, and an MA in Jewish studies and PhD in social ethics from the Graduate Theological Union in Berkeley.

Leonard I. Zon, MD, is professor of pediatrics and a Howard Hughes Medical Institute investigator at Children's Hospital in Boston. He received a BS in chemistry and natural sciences from Muhlenberg College and an MD from Jefferson Medical College. He did an internal medicine residency at New England Deaconess Hospital and a fellowship in medical oncology at Dana-Farber Cancer Institute. His postdoctoral research was in the laboratory of Stuart Orkin. Dr. Zon's research focuses on the zebrafish, a new genetic and developmental model system for understanding blood formation. His laboratory has characterized over 26 mutant groups that can live with decreased blood or no blood at all. Several of them represent models of human disease. Dr. Zon is the president of the International Society for Stem Cell Research.

Index

A

Abnormalities, found in cloned animals, 34
Accountability issues, 51
Adult stem cells, 17, 115
Advanced Cell Technology, 15
Alzheimer's disease, 33
American Society for Reproductive Medicine (ASRM), 27
    Ethics Committee, 27, 52
American Type Culture Collection, 93
Androgenesis, 37, 100, 103, 115
    diploid androgenetic mES cells, 36
Animal care and use, 70–71
    handling chimeras with human-like characteristics, 50
Animal cells, mixing with, disclosure that cells and cell lines could be used in, 91, 102, 127
Animal feeder cells, 18
Animal Welfare Act, 71
ART. *See* Assisted reproductive technology
Asilomar Conference, 26–27, 70
ASRM. *See* American Society for Reproductive Medicine
Assisted human reproduction agency, in Canada, 27
Assisted reproductive technology (ART), 81, 91–92
    services offering, 10

Australia, 76–77
    national body established in, 59
    procurement practices in, 66
Authorizations, 68–69, 126
Autologous transplantation, 9, 34, 44, 84, 115
Autonomy, 9, 58, 85, 101

B

Banking and distribution of hES cell lines, 92–95, 103–105
    facilities for implementing specific recommended standards, 94–95, 104–105, 129–130
    institutions establishing uniform guidelines and record-keeping processes approved by an IRB, 94, 103–104, 128
    recommendations for, 12–13
Benefits
    of hES cell research, just distribution of, 60
    personal, informing donors there will be none, 9, 84
Best Practices for the Licensing of Genomic Inventions, 64
Bioethics Advisory Committee
    in Israel, 78
    in Singapore, 78
Biohazards, 59